FREE
Yourself
from
Chronic
Pain
and ***Sports Injuries***

FREE
Yourself
from
Chronic
Pain
and **Sports Injuries**

How Prolotherapy Can
Help You Become Pain Free

Donna Alderman, D.O.
Osteopathic Physician and Surgeon

FAMILY DOCTOR
PRESS

Glendale, CA

Free Yourself from Chronic Pain and Sports Injuries
Copyright © 2008 by Donna Alderman, D.O.

Family Doctor Press
1740 Broadview Drive
Glendale, CA 91208
www.familydoctorpress.com

This book is for educational purposes. It is not intended as a substitute for medical advice. Please consult a qualified health care professional for individual health and medical advice. Neither the publisher nor the author shall have any responsibility for any adverse effects arising directly or indirectly as a result of the information provided in this book.

Publisher's Cataloging-In-Publication Data

Alderman, Donna.
   Free yourself from chronic pain and sports injuries : how prolotherapy can help you become pain free / Donna Alderman.

    p. ; cm.

   Includes bibliographical references and index.
   ISBN-13: 978-0-9815242-0-7
   ISBN-10: 0-9815242-0-6

1. Chronic pain--Treatment. 2. Chronic pain--Alternative treatment. 3. Sports injuries--Treatment. 4. Sports injuries--Alternative treatment. I. Title.

RB127 .A43 2008
616/.0472
2008900984

Book and cover designer: Pamela Terry, Opus 1 Design, www.opus1design.com
Book Consultant: Brookes Nohlgren, www.booksbybrookes.com

Printed in the United States of America on acid-free paper

This book is dedicated to
Gustav Hemwall, M.D. (1908–1998),
a pioneer in Prolotherapy, for his work
in the field and for his courage
to explore new ways to help his patients.

I would also like to dedicate this book
to the wonderful patients I have had over
the years, from whom I have learned so much.

Contents

Disclaimer

The information presented in this book is based on the experiences of Donna Alderman, D.O., and is for educational and informational purposes only. In no way should this book be used as a substitute for your own physician's advice. It is sold with the understanding that the publisher and author are not engaged in rendering medical or other professional services, and does not constitute a doctor-patient relationship. Do not rely upon the information in this book without seeking independent professional medical advice.

Prolotherapy is a medical technique. As with any medical technique, it may not be right for you and results will vary among individuals. Prolotherapy may not work for you, and as with all medical procedures there are risks involved. These risks should be discussed with a qualified healthcare professional prior to any treatment.

Physicians should use and apply the technique of Prolotherapy only after they have received extensive training and demonstrated the ability to safely administer the treatment. The author, publisher, and publishing agent are not responsible if physicians who are unqualified in the use of Prolotherapy administer the treatment based solely on the contents of this book. The author and publisher shall have neither liability nor responsibility to any person or entity with respect to any loss or damage caused or alleged to be caused directly or indirectly by the information contained in this book.

Patient stories in this book are intended to inform, educate, and entertain. Responses to any medical treatment are individual, and results vary among individuals. There is no guarantee that you or anyone else will receive the same outcome. If Prolotherapy appears to apply to your condition, the author recommends that a formal evaluation be performed by a physician who is competent in treating chronic pain with Prolotherapy. Those desiring treatment should make medical decisions with the aid of a personal physician. No medical decisions should be based solely on the contents or recommendations made in this book.

FOREWORD

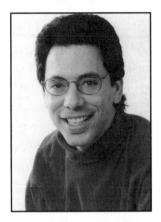

Ross A. Hauser, M.D.

The consummate physician will do what is best for the patient, no matter the circumstance. For those physicians who dare tackle the chronic pain patient, this means getting involved in the treatment known as Prolotherapy. I was fortunate enough to write one of the books on the subject, *Prolo Your Pain Away!*, and as I promoted this book I was able to meet some of the doctors around the country who were utilizing this technique. At an American College for the Advancement of Medicine meeting in the early 1990s, I first came across the enthusiasm and energy of Dr. Donna Alderman. When Dr. Alderman saw my table and book, she cried out, "I love Prolotherapy! I just learned it and it's wonderful!" She immediately grabbed up several copies of my book, and a bond of friendship was struck between us. She received additional training in Prolotherapy, by the grandmaster Dr. Gustav Hemwall, and was a volunteer at Beulah Land Natural

Medicine Clinic in rural Illinois, utilizing her skills as a Prolotherapist to relieve the chronic pain and suffering of so many people. Not only have I had the opportunity to help train Dr. Alderman, but have also been fortunate enough to work beside her and see her compassion for the patient and passion for Prolotherapy.

Dr. Alderman is the consummate physician in her desire to get at the root cause of the patient's problems. As it relates to chronic pain she has found, as have her natural medicine colleagues, that the treatment that gives the most lasting results is Prolotherapy. Dr. Alderman has discovered, as I have, that nothing gives faster, more lasting results for the chronic pain sufferer than Prolotherapy.

Dr. Alderman has utilized her interest for Prolotherapy in a most important way by putting her knowledge into the book *Free Yourself from Chronic Pain and Sports Injuries: How Prolotherapy Can Help You Become Pain Free*, in which she explains in easy-to-understand language the central tenets of Prolotherapy. She goes through her own story and why, even as a Doctor of Osteopathic Medicine, she did not have the entire answer to her patients' chronic pain complaints until she herself learned and performed Prolotherapy. She goes through why ligament and tendon weakness is the most common cause for musculoskeletal chronic pain, why these structures don't heal, and finally how Prolotherapy can cause these structures to strengthen. She goes into detail as to the *hows, whys,* and *whats* about the fact that Prolotherapy stimulates the body to repair painful areas.

You do not need to know anything about medicine to read Dr. Alderman's book. She understands that as people search the Internet in the hope of finding a cure for their chronic pain, they will need resources. One of the best resources they will find is Dr. Alderman's book on Prolotherapy. In it, people will find wonderful case histories including how Dr. Alderman helped even skeptics like her mother get over their chronic pain, and stories of famous people such as John Gray, author of *Men Are from Mars, Woman Are from Venus,* who have been set free from chronic pain by Prolotherapy. John Gray notes, "After just one Prolotherapy treatment I felt immediate improvement. After five treatments, my neck is fantastic and I am virtually pain-free. My posture has improved, and I feel stronger. I no longer have low back pain, the pain down my leg is gone, and my ankle has more bounce and doesn't click like it used to." **John Gray's response is not unique; it is typical of people who receive Prolotherapy.**

Free Yourself from Chronic Pain and Sports Injuries explains how Prolotherapy can eliminate pain in the neck, back, ankles, and other parts of the body. It shows how Prolotherapy can even relieve the pain of herniated discs, arthritis, degenerated joints and discs, tendonosis (degenerated tendons), ligament sprains, tendon strains, and sports injuries.

So you have chronic pain and want to be free of it? What are you going to do? Dr. Alderman puts it best when she says, "Life is full of choices. Granted, you may not have chosen to be in a motor vehicle accident that left you with years of neck and back pain, or while playing basketball to twist an ankle that never quite healed. *But you can choose what to do about it.*"

It is my hope that by reading this book you will come to the same conclusion as Dr. Alderman. She has learned, as you will by reading her book, that there is a way to set yourself free from chronic pain—and that way is Prolotherapy.

Ross A. Hauser, M.D.
Author of *Prolo Your Pain Away!*

Dr. Ross Hauser earned his medical degree from the University of Illinois. He went on to receive specialty training in Physical Medicine and Rehabilitation. His desire to be a chronic pain specialist led him to join the practice of Gustav Hemwall, M.D., one of the foremost authorities on Prolotherapy. At Caring Medical and Rehabilitation Services in Oak Park, Illinois, Dr. Hauser uses Prolotherapy in treating chronic pain. Dr. Hauser and his wife, Marion, have written eight books on Prolotherapy, including *Prolo Your Pain Away!* and *Prolo Your Sports Injuries Away!*

PREFACE

WHY PROLOTHERAPY?

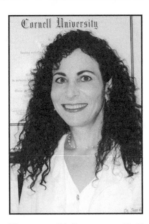

Donna Alderman, D.O.

When a person becomes a physician, he or she learns the Hippocratic Oath, which sets down the rules for practicing medicine. The first and foremost rule of this doctrine is "to help, or at least, do no harm." Musculoskeletal pain—such as low back or neck pain; elbow, shoulder, or wrist pain; ankle, foot, or knee pain; and other joint pain—is a common complaint heard by many a family physician. As a young doctor practicing family medicine, I had patient after patient come to me with these ailments.

Being an osteopathic physician, with extra training in the musculoskeletal system and treatment, I probably knew more than the average medical doctor regarding these issues. However, for some of my patients, their pain persisted. Because of my belief that a doctor should "do no harm," I was reluctant to prescribe long-term painkillers, which have potential side effects and can be addictive, or to send someone for an invasive procedure such as surgery, unless the need was clear-cut, which is rare. I was getting discouraged. Yet, I did not give up. With all that medical science had to offer, I thought there must be *something* I could do to help these patients. Then I heard about Prolotherapy.

Prolotherapy is a minimally invasive, safe therapy that stimulates the body to heal painful areas. It has a high success rate and strengthens tissue rather than weakening it, as can happen with other treatments such as cortisone. My goal in writing this book is to provide factual information about Prolotherapy and to share my experiences with it. My hope is to educate in a fun, easy way. After all, *doctor* comes from a Latin word meaning "teacher," and an important part of a doctor's job is to educate and inform. Thanks to the Internet, where a vast amount of information is now available at our fingertips, our society is shifting to one where patients do their own research and take a more active role in making decisions about their medical treatments. The more patients know about their options, the better equipped they will be to make informed choices that are right for them. While Prolotherapy is not for everyone or for every condition, it has helped thousands of people who might otherwise still be in pain.

ACKNOWLEDGMENTS

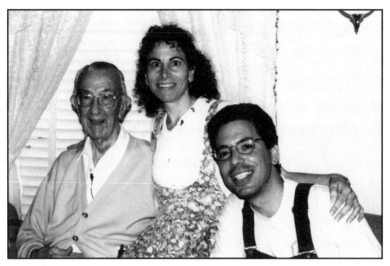

Dr. Alderman (center) with Dr. Gustav Hemwall (left) and Dr. Ross Hauser (right) at the First Annual Prolotherapy Training Seminar in Thebes, Illinois

When I first heard about Prolotherapy, I thought, "This is too good to be true—a natural, non-surgical treatment for chronic pain!" But, I discovered, it was true. Had it not been for my instructors in Prolotherapy, I would not have made it to this point. I want to thank Ross Hauser, M.D., who generously shared his time and expertise in mentoring me and who showed me that a doctor can be funny, smart, caring, and athletic (he has completed the Iron Man competition!). I also want to thank Gustav Hemwall, M.D., who was known as "the world's most experienced Prolotherapist" until he passed away in 1998, and who provided inspiration for my continued studies. I want to thank Tom Raven, M.D.; Tom

Cantieri, D.O.; and George Pasquarello, D.O.; instructors at the University of New England School of Osteopathic Medicine course in Prolotherapy, for their patience and dedication. Thanks also go to William Faber, D.O., of the Milwaukee Pain Clinic, for introducing me to this wonderful treatment. I also want to thank my mother, Bess Alderman, R.N., who provided love and a positive attitude through all my endeavors (although she used to call Prolotherapy "voodoo"— that is, until I fixed her knee!). And, finally, I want to thank my friend Craig, who turned me from a sports illiterate into an avid basketball fan and who taught me the importance of not dwelling on a missed pass or basket, but staying alert and productive because the ball may be coming back to you at any moment.

Free Yourself *from* Chronic Pain *and Sports Injuries*

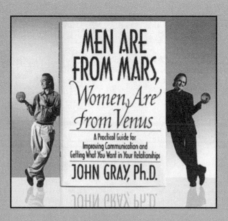

A Writer

After 25 years as a professional writer and many hours at the computer, my neck and back were beginning to feel like a pretzel. The frequent traveling I do didn't help, and I often felt as if my neck was in a tight vise. My posture was worsening and I began to get low back pain, sometimes with sciatic nerve pain down my leg. My ankle, as well, had been bothering me for over 10 years, a consequence of aggressive physical activity in my youth. Over the years I had tried chiropractic and acupuncture, but I was still in pain and it wasn't getting any better. Then, through a friend, I heard about Prolotherapy.

After just one Prolotherapy treatment, I felt immediate improvement. After five treatments, my neck is fantastic and I am virtually pain free. My posture has improved, and I feel stronger. I no longer have low back pain, the pain down my leg is gone, and my ankle has more bounce and doesn't click like it used to.

Prolotherapy is something you can do to take control of the downward spiral of aging and chronic pain. You have the power to do something positive to improve your physical condition, without drugs, without surgery. It worked for me.

John Gray, Ph.D.
Author of *Men Are from Mars, Woman Are from Venus*

CHAPTER 1

M.D.s and D.O.s:
What's the Difference?

Before going further, I want to address the question of what kind of doctor I am. Many times over the years I have been asked, "What is a D.O.?" This is a fair question. I have been referred to as an "M.D." and while I am a *medical doctor*, licensed to practice full general medicine, to use the term "M.D." is technically incorrect. Therefore, I'd like to set the record straight and also provide an interesting bit of history about the practice of medicine in the United States. What you are about to read will almost certainly make you a more informed consumer of U.S. medical care.

Many people do not know that there are two types of fully licensed medical doctors in the United States—one receives an M.D. degree, "Medical Doctor," and the other receives a D.O. degree, "Doctor of Osteopathic Medicine." For each, the license to practice medicine is equivalent.

One of the largest medical insurance companies in the U.S. states in the "DEFINITIONS" section of its policies:

"DOCTOR OF MEDICINE: a licensed medical doctor (M.D.) or doctor of osteopathic medicine (D.O.)."[1]

The Business and Professions Code for the State of California (where I practice) states:

"M.D. and D.O. Degrees - Equal Status: It is the policy of this state that holders of M.D. degrees and D.O. degrees shall be accorded equal professional status and privileges as licensed physicians and surgeons."[2]

Medical school education for M.D.s and D.O.s is equivalent, with the exception that D.O.s not only receive training in pharmacology (prescribing medication), basic medicine, and surgery, but also receive extra training in the musculoskeletal system, a vital component of the human body. Like an M.D., a D.O. can specialize after basic medical training is completed, and become, for instance, a dermatologist, surgeon, pediatrician, gynecologist, or any other specialty. So why have two separate degrees for what would appear to be the same thing? To understand this, we need to look at the history of medicine in this country.

A hundred and fifty years ago, medicine was barbaric. Bloodletting, arsenic, and mercury "treatments" were the mainstay of medical doctors. Dr. Andrew Still, an M.D. practicing in the 1800s, stood by and helplessly watched his young children die of meningitis. This traumatic event was a turning point for Dr. Still. For the next 10 years, he studied the human body and better ways to treat disease.

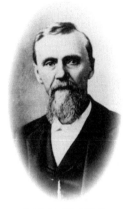

A.T. Still, M.D.
1828–1917

"Seek Health in Your Patients, Any Fool Can Find Disease."[3] This was Dr. Still's philosophy. Dr. Still was a critic of using the day's harsh drugs and therapeutic remedies such as bloodletting (opening a vein and letting it bleed to get rid of disease), or using mercury, lead, and arsenic, which were often ineffective and sometimes harmful. He strongly believed that if a body was put in correct alignment, given good nutrition, and if circulation was improved, the body could better heal itself. He believed that the physician's role was to assist the patient to a healthier condition, not to be a dictator of prescribed remedies. Dr. Still stressed preventive medicine, good nutrition, and the importance of the musculoskeletal system, including correct alignment of the bones (hence the term *osteopathic*: *osteo* from Latin, meaning "bone," and *pathic* from Greek, meaning "suffering"), as well as muscle balance and improved nerve, lymph, and blood flow to enhance the body's natural healing ability.

Dr. Still's philosophy became the School of Osteopathy, now known as *Osteopathic Medicine*, named after its original emphasis on the musculoskeletal system. Osteopathic medicine went on to father physical medicine and rehabilitation, physical therapy, and the Western healing arts that involve using hands to improve body mobility and function.

As Western medical science advanced with the development of the germ theory and the discovery of antibiotics, osteopathic medicine followed suit, providing education to its students in medicine and surgery as well as osteopathic treatment. Today, both M.D. and D.O. medical school programs are nearly identical—with the same intense coursework—except that D.O. medical students are required to take additional coursework that covers the musculoskeletal system, physical medicine, and osteopathic philosophical principles. Medical residency programs are mixed with D.O.s and M.D.s working alongside each other, and in many specialties Board certification exams are the same for both D.O.s and M.D.s. Therefore, the term *osteopathic* has a philosophical origin but, for the modern D.O., is a bit of a misnomer because today's D.O. is a complete medical doctor, with the added benefit of this extra training.

In California, many people are unfamiliar with the D.O. degree. This is, in part, because of a political event that occurred in California over 40 years ago. By the 1960s, the standards of practice for D.O.s and M.D.s had grown very close together. The sentiment was growing among some D.O.s and M.D.s that the two professions should unite. Therefore, the M.D.s and D.O.s constructed an agreement such that for a minimal trade-in fee, a D.O. could send in his or her diploma and get an M.D. diploma. While this may have eliminated some confusion for the general public in choosing a doctor, it was a step backward for the osteopathic profession in California. Thousands of D.O.s simply "vanished" behind M.D. degrees, where their special talents and extra training could not be openly appreciated. In other parts of the country where no such political event occurred, osteopathic medicine is better understood. In fact, there are many osteopathic hospitals in the Midwest and on the East Coast.

I chose osteopathic medicine because it aligns with my own concept of healthcare: embracing preventive medicine and nutrition, where the doctor and patient work together toward the common goal of excellent health. And, of course, being an osteopathic physician has given me tremendous insight into the musculoskeletal system, and ultimately led me to Prolotherapy. Now, more about Prolotherapy!

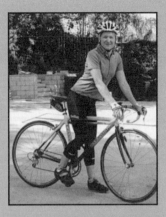

An Active Housewife

I have always led a very active life and consider exercise to be my biggest "hobby." I am 46 years old and have enjoyed biking, running, yoga, Pilates, hiking, yard work, and basically anything physical. Up until 2004, I never had any chronic ailment or pain that limited me in any way.

In March 2004, I noticed an area around my back and hip that was tender, with increasing discomfort and pain. I had been running a lot, so I cut back. Still, the pain became worse, so I saw a chiropractor who diagnosed me with a hip flexor problem, which he said was common in runners. I received electrical stimulation and ultrasound, but the problem continued to intensify dramatically. It felt as if a nerve had become irritated, and I resorted to all kinds of pain medication.

The pain became so unbearable that I was eventually admitted to a hospital for pain control. While there for six days, I had a complete workup—MRIs, x-rays, and so on—but they could not find anything wrong. I received cortisone shots and physical therapy, which did little or nothing to help me.

For the next six months, I continued to need more and more pain medication and started to have sleep difficulties. I saw four doctors, all of whom had different opinions about the cause of my pain. In short, I was told I would need to live with it, take pain medications, and probably eventually need a spinal fusion. I was devastated. I was so sick of medication and the way it made me feel, and desperate to get back to doing even simple household chores. Walking around the block was about all I could muster.

I had almost given up hope that I could someday be active again when a friend told me about Prolotherapy and how it had helped her. In reading about Prolotherapy, I found that it was pretty much the opposite of everything I had been doing. It sounded so logical, with little downside. My first visit with Dr. Alderman was great. She, unlike the other doctors I had seen, took the time to hear my story and seemed to integrate all the information, and I started treatment.

I have really had remarkable results with Prolotherapy. Over a period of months, I sensed an increased strength/mobility in my back. I have been able to resume almost all of the activities I used to enjoy, and am now close to 100 percent better. I have told everybody I know about Prolotherapy. Prolotherapy got me off pain medication, helped take away my pain, and has given me the ability to be active again and enjoy a very physical life.

Jane Edwards
Housewife

CHAPTER 2

Prolotherapy Basics

Prolotherapy is based on a very simple principle: **the body has the capacity to heal itself.** This is not a foreign concept. Think about this example: You get a paper cut. You first notice there is a rip in your skin and a little blood. Then, the wound stops bleeding, is a little red and sore where the cut occurred, and within a few days the skin is healed. This is a stimulus-response system: you injure yourself (stimulus), and that sets into motion a cascade of actions that result in healing (response). A healthy body routinely and automatically responds this way, healing itself if it can.

With musculoskeletal injuries, a similar "stimulus-response" occurs. However, the healing time is much longer than with a simple paper cut—weeks to months rather than days. Another difference is that even in a healthy person, the body has a tendency not to heal 100 percent from ligament and tendon injuries. To understand why this occurs, and how Prolotherapy can help, it is important to understand a little bit about the body's composition. Here is what I call my "PROLOTHERAPY 101" lecture:

Look at this picture of the shoulder joint. The white part of the muscle, which attaches it to the joint, is the *tendon*. Bones are connected to bones by *ligaments*. Ligaments and tendons are known as *connective tissue* because they connect the joints of the body together.

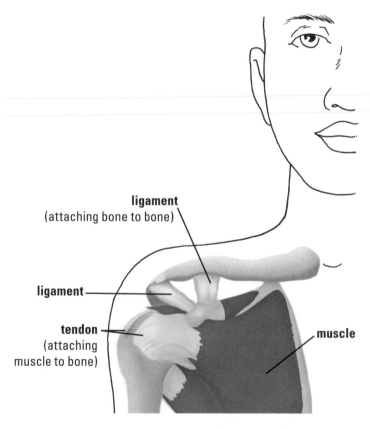

FIGURE 2–1: **The Shoulder Joint**

QUESTION: Notice that the muscle is red; however, the tendon portion, which attaches the muscle to the bone, is a whitish color. Also note that ligaments (connecting bone to bone) are also whitish in color. Why do you think muscles are red and ligaments and tendons are white? What is present in large amounts in muscle that makes it appear red, but only present in small amounts in ligaments and tendons?

ANSWER: Blood!

There is only a small blood supply in ligaments and tendons. This means slow healing, even under the best of circumstances. Injuries to ligaments and tendons can take weeks to months to heal. A typical ligament or tendon injury takes four to six weeks to heal, with the most healing occurring in the first two weeks after an injury.

Unfortunately, after the typical four- to six-week healing cycle is over, the body's stimulus to heal has significantly diminished. In other words, if healing does not occur within the first month or so after an injury, it is not likely to occur later on its own. To further complicate the healing issue, even under the best of circumstances connective tissue may not heal 100 percent on its own.

In fact, it has been estimated that the usual best result of a connective tissue repair cycle may be as little as 50–60 percent of pre-injury strength.[1] Each time a joint is injured, the risk exists that it will not heal completely. And if the injury does not heal completely—

even if it heals 95 percent each time rather than 100 percent—the ligaments and/or tendons of that joint become a little weaker and more predisposed to another injury. Recurrent injury to the same joint, followed by that joint's failure to heal completely, may occur over and over again, each time reducing the area's overall strength and stability and causing pain. If this occurs enough times, weakness and pain become chronic (i.e., the pain does not go away).

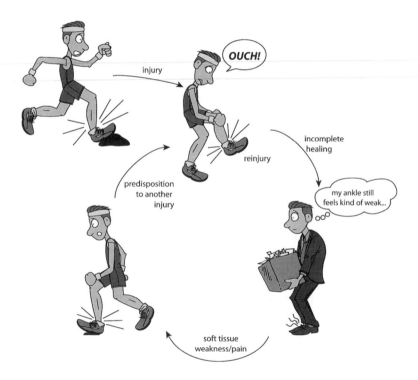

FIGURE 2–2: **Vicious Cycle of Soft Tissue Injury**

Ligaments and tendons are composed of collagen—a very strong protein—and other fibers, designed to give strength and some, limited, flexibility. However, when overstretched—such as might occur with lifting a heavy object, turning in the wrong direction, or even small repetitive trauma—these tissues may sustain tears or micro-tears. Ligaments and tendons do not just "bounce back." They must heal back. If the tear is too large, or if the tendon or ligament has been pulled off the bone, surgery may be needed. However, in most cases the ligament or tendon does not pull off the bone but simply becomes lax (overstretched) and sustains small tears. Even small micro-tears can cause significant pain and weakness if they do not heal.

In repetitive strain, where small, minor repetitive movements can, over time, result in a larger problem, each individual small injury may not be sufficient to provide enough stimulus to promote complete healing. In those cases, even minor injury may be enough to accumulate damage to the point of initiating chronic pain.[2]

Unfortunately, the occurrence of chronic pain may eventually impair the activities of an otherwise active person. It can be slow and progressive, until one day the individual finds he or she can no longer do the desired activity or sport without pain, and may even give it up. Here is an example of what can happen:

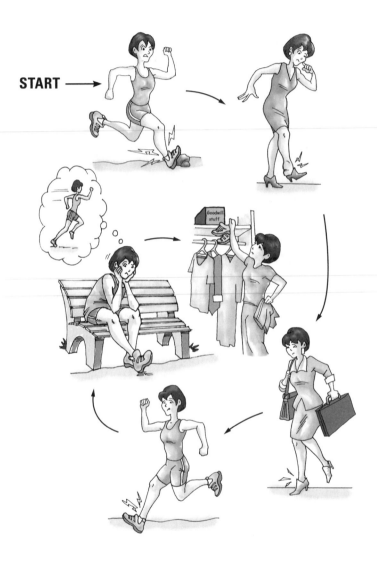

FIGURE 2–3

EXAMPLE: Alice is running one morning and sprains her ankle. What is the first thing that occurs?

In the body's attempt to get blood to the injured area, the ankle swells dramatically. Alice is upset, not only because the ankle hurts, but also because she is now limping and can't fit into her new shoes. The ankle continues to be swollen for a few weeks, then the swelling gradually decreases over the next four to six weeks. Alice can wear her shoes now, but the ankle still hurts a little. She had previous injuries to the ankle, but seemed to always recover from these injuries after a few weeks and never noticed a problem that lasted. However, each injury and subsequent injury did weaken her ankle. This time Alice notices a low-level, constant pain and a feeling of weakness in her ankle that doesn't go away after the six-week healing cycle. This last injury was the "straw that broke the camel's back." Alice eventually gives up running.

How Does Prolotherapy Help?

Prolotherapy creates an effective stimulus that causes the body to respond with its own natural healing cycle. It does this by "tricking" the body into healing by creating a directed, local irritation and temporary inflammation at the site of the injury. This, then, stimulates the body to send blood and repair cells as well as to increase the activity of growth factors to make new collagen and repair the weak and painful areas. That is why Prolotherapy can help years after the injury, pain, or weakness first occurred. Prolotherapy provides a very directed stimulus to the specific sites where the original injury occurred. In this way, Prolotherapy creates a controlled, concentrated "stimulus-response" healing cycle to areas that otherwise would not be stimulated to heal on their own.

Prolotherapy is short for *proliferation therapy*, named so because it stimulates the proliferation (growth) and re-generation of injured ligaments and tendons by increasing blood flow and activating production of growth factors,[3] proteins that stimulate tissue repair and growth. Tissue biopsies of ligaments and/or tendons treated with Prolotherapy have demonstrated increased texture and strength in multiple studies.[4, 5, 6, 7] And although not studied in humans, growth factor stimulation in animals has shown repair of full thickness cartilage defects in injection studies.[8,9]

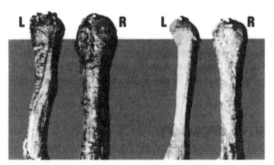

9 months   12 months

FIGURE 2–4: **Photograph of Rabbit Tendons at Nine and Twelve Months After Three Injections of Proliferating Solution into the Right Tendons**
Reproduced by permission from Ross A. Hauser and Marion A. Hauser, *Prolo Your Pain Away!* (Oak Park, IL: Beulah Land Press, 2004), 34.

Prolotherapy has been endorsed by C. Everett Koop, M.D., the former United States Surgeon General,[10] and has been practiced in the U.S. for over 50 years. It has a high success rate, low risk, and few side effects. The principle of Prolotherapy is simple...as Dr. Hemwall said at a conference one year, "too simple." Simple or not, Prolotherapy has a high success rate in helping injured and weak ligaments and tendons heal and regain strength, reducing or eliminating pain. So how does Prolotherapy do this? Read on!

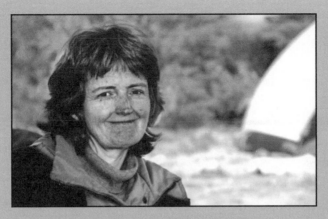

An Environmental Inspector

My work involves walking and hiking in outdoor terrain. About three years ago, I started to have crippling, chronic pain in my lower legs and was diagnosed with "shin splints." I saw a podiatrist who gave me orthotics, which did not help. I also saw an orthopedic surgeon who prescribed months of very strong anti-inflammatories and stretching exercises, which helped only a very small amount. I still could not walk without being in significant pain. I also saw a sports medicine doctor who did a bone scan, which was normal, and put me on anti-inflammatories, which did not help. The pain became chronic and would flare as soon as I started to walk. It became so painful that it would wake me up at night. During the day, I was limping in pain with each step. I was having trouble doing the walking involved in my job and was desperate to find a solution to my problem.

Then I found out about Prolotherapy and began receiving treatments to my ankles and knees, and am now virtually pain free. I am amazingly better, and able to do my job, including hiking, without pain. Each week I continue to feel stronger. I am very grateful for this simple, but incredibly effective, treatment and to Dr. Alderman.

Antonia Lattin
Environmental Inspector

CHAPTER 3

Causes of Chronic Musculoskeletal Pain and Why Prolotherapy Works

As we've just discussed, ligament and tendon weakness (also called "relaxation" or "laxity") is a common cause of chronic musculoskeletal pain,[1] and it is this problem that Prolotherapy addresses. What does that mean exactly? When injury or trauma occurs to a ligament that holds a joint together, the result can be overstretching or micro-tearing of that ligament. The joint becomes loose, which leads to instability, weakness, and pain. Similarly, any tendon throughout the body can become chronically relaxed and thus a source of pain.[2] Whether tendon or ligament, if proper healing does not occur, joint instability and pain result.[3] As early as the 1950s, some physicians recognized the potential of this treatment for strengthening ligaments and stabilizing joints.[4]

Even disc herniations have been linked to ligament weakness. As early as 1952, it was observed that weakness of the ligaments around the spine came *before* disc herniations, sometimes years before the actual disc herniations occurred.[5] Dr. P.H. Newman, a British surgeon in the 1950s with years of experience performing disc operations, concluded that torn or inefficient spinal ligaments resulted in unstable vertebrae and preceded disc herniations.[6] He believed the most common cause of chronic low back pain was a strain on a segment of the spine that occurred *after* the ligaments had already been injured.[7]

Ligament or tendon weakness may occur due to a known accident, injury, or trauma, such as a motor vehicle accident or sports injury, but can also happen as a result of smaller, repetitive traumas that are not as obvious a source. This type of injury, which frequently "sneaks up on" a person, is common, for example, in someone who uses a body part repetitively, such as a mechanic who twists his arm to turn a wrench, a warehouse worker who regularly lifts boxes, or a student or office worker who sits at a computer day after day. Ligament or tendon weakness can also sneak up on athletes who repeatedly injure themselves, and may also appear in someone without any known history of injury.

In athletes, joint injuries are common. Usually a player with a serious ligament or tendon injury is put on the "injured list" and not allowed to play until healed. However, even when a player has healed enough to get back into the game, the injured area may not be truly

100 percent and thus is more susceptible to another injury. Additionally, an athlete may not report or even notice smaller injuries and so may continue to play on an injured or weakened joint. Repetitive strain is also a factor. A basketball player who jumps over and over again with a back that eventually begins to hurt or on an ankle that is repeatedly sprained can accumulate small injuries until one final injury becomes the "straw that breaks the camel's back," resulting in pain that doesn't go away.

BIOMECHANICS CHANGE WHEN A JOINT IS INJURED

Increased relaxation (excess motion) of a joint results not only in that joint's instability, but also a change in its biomechanics. Biomechanics is the study of the action of forces and motion ("mechanics") on a living body ("bio"). An injured joint puts extra stress on other joints in that body, which can eventually result in more areas of pain. For instance, if a person injures his or her knee, it is likely that person will alter the way he or she walks in order to decrease the injury's pain or discomfort. Over time, even a slight change in one's walk may have an impact, for example, on the knee cartilage or on the hip, foot, or back. As the body compensates for the injury—taking the stress off that injured joint by instead using other joints or body areas—the result can be a domino effect where other joints then begin to become painful.

Therefore, as you can see, it is important that joints be stable and strong. Illustrating this point further is a condition known as "hypermobility," where a person's joints have the tendency to overstretch and therefore may be more prone to injury and pain. An extreme example of what can happen when joints are unstable is a class of connective tissue diseases where ligaments and tendons are genetically too elastic and too flexible, resulting in chronically dislocating joints. The worst of these is Ehlers-Danlos Syndrome (named after the doctors who discovered it). People with Ehlers-Danlos live a painful, difficult existence. Many of their joints regularly or constantly dislocate, making even life's ordinary activities very challenging. Often, individuals with Ehlers-Danlos need multiple joint surgeries over the course of their lifetime just to be able to use their joints and function normally. While this is an extreme example, you can see that even a milder version of joint instability, such as an unhealed overstretched ligament, can cause problems with joint function and pain.

MUSCLE SPASM FOLLOWS JOINT INJURY

Increased joint motion (instability) stimulates the body to want to "fix" the problem. Even a small amount of excess motion in a joint can trigger this response. Nearby muscles will tighten, creating muscle spasm, in an attempt to stabilize the loose joint. However, muscles were not designed to do the job of the ligament, and eventually they fatigue. If this muscle spasm continues for too long, the muscles may develop "trigger points"—areas of perpetual tightening. These trigger points can be felt as muscle knots, which are sore and tender to the touch (they "trigger" pain). Thus, the body's attempt to fix the initial problem creates another problem: chronic muscular tightness and spasm!

Osteoarthritis Is Next

Osteoarthritis is the sometimes painful condition where bony deposits form in a joint. Also known as "degenerative arthritis," it is often diagnosed from an x-ray, where these findings can easily be seen. Many people have these type of deposits on x-ray, yet do not have any symptoms or problems. However, in some people osteoarthritis bony overgrowth and degeneration can cause problems such as restricted movement and pain.[8]

There are various theories of how osteoarthritis develops. In the medical literature, there is a clear relationship between ligament and tendon injury and later development of osteoarthritis.

To demonstrate how and why this might happen, let's take a theoretical person, Joe, who was in a car accident and suffered a whiplash. Whiplash is an injury that snaps the neck backward and forward, stretching out the neck ligaments. Joe's neck is sore and tender after the accident and the muscles around his neck become tight. This is his body's attempt to "solve" the problem of joint instability—his muscles become tight in an effort to stabilize the now loose and overstretched ligaments and tendons in his neck. Unfortunately, because muscles were not intended to support joints, this "solution" doesn't work well. Further, because Joe is now less active than he used to be before his accident, over time his muscles may atrophy (become smaller and weaker), making them even less capable of holding his weakened neck.

Because the body's solution of muscle tightening is not truly curing the problem, after a while if the joint has not healed, the body goes to "Plan B." Being very clever indeed, over many years the body starts depositing something in the neck joints to help restrict the excess motion caused by the overstretched, unhealed ligaments and/or tendons. Can you guess what that something is? You got it … calcium! Remember that bony spurs and calcium deposits in a joint is a condition known as osteoarthritis, the most common form of arthritis.

What is the medical evidence for this theory? One study of female soccer players who had sustained knee ligament injury showed a very high percentage with knee osteoarthritis 12 years later.[9] Another study, published in *Sports Medicine*, observed the increased incidence of arthritis with individuals who engaged in certain sports, for instance wrestlers, boxers, baseball pitchers, football players, ballet dancers, soccer players, weightlifters, cricket players, and gymnasts.[10]

In veterinary medicine, it is well established that ligament sprains favor the development of osteoarthritis in animals.[11] A well-known medical journal reports:

> "There is no question that trauma and mechanical stress on the joint lead to the development of osteoarthritis."[12]

This logic is further supported by Wolff's Law (named after Dr. Julius Wolff, who reported it): "Bones respond to stress by making new bone."[13] A change in biomechanics brought about by the ligament or tendon injury puts stress on the joint, which then responds to that stress by laying down more bone. This can be seen in Figure 3-1, on the following page:

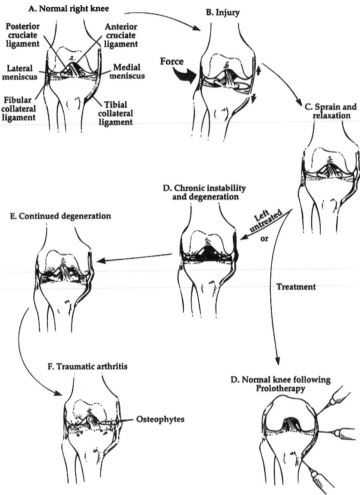

FIGURE 3-1: **How Soft Tissue Injury Leads to Degenerative Arthritis**
Ligaments become sprained following trauma. When healing does not
occur, the ligaments become relaxed, resulting in chronic instability
and degeneration from meniscal and articular cartilage degeneration.
When left untreated, post-traumatic "arthritis" or degenerative osteoarthritis follows. This degenerative process can be prevented with appropriate intervention through Prolotherapy.

Reproduced by permission from Ross A. Hauser and Marion A. Hauser, *Prolo
Your Pain Away!* (Oak Park, IL: Beulah Land Press, 2004), 134.

Prolotherapy has been shown to be effective at treating musculoskeletal pain caused by osteoarthritis.[14, 15, 16] The most likely reason for this is that Prolotherapy treats the reason the arthritis developed: joint instability. However, the bony spurs themselves do not go away (remember, they took years to develop). While Prolotherapy is still a treatment option even after someone has developed osteoarthritis, it is of course better to treat joint instability before osteoarthritis has developed or at least before it has become severe.

WHY DOESN'T THE LIGAMENT OR TENDON TISSUE HEAL ON ITS OWN IN THE FIRST PLACE?

As you may remember from "Prolotherapy 101" in Chapter 2, injuries involving ligaments and tendons are slow to heal because the blood supply to those areas is poor. Blood is a powerful healing agent because it carries growth factors that help to regenerate injured tissue. Lifestyle factors such as poor nutrition, poor-quality sleep, smoking, certain medications, or continuing to overuse an injured joint may prevent complete healing.

Important to healing is the rebuilding of collagen—a strong, fibrous, insoluble protein that is a major component of ligament and tendon tissue. The word *collagen* comes from the Greek *kola*, meaning "glue," and *gennan*, meaning "to produce."[17] This strong, glue-like protein is critical to healing an injured ligament or tendon.

Various factors reduce or prevent collagen repair. Poor nutrition is one. For example, without vitamin C the body cannot properly rebuild collagen. In fact, scurvy, a disease common in sailors in the 1800s, is an extreme example of vitamin C deficiency. In scurvy, lack of vitamin C prevents normal collagen repair, resulting in fatigue and joint pain. The sailors' diet in those days lacked fruits, and by adding a lime, lemon, or orange daily the problem was solved.

Another factor affecting healing is sleep. Sleep is important for regenerating normal day-to-day injuries. This is because, while sleeping, the body makes growth hormone, which stimulates the repair of collagen and other tissues. If a person is under stress and not sleeping well, he or she will not heal as effectively. Normal day-to-day micro-injuries to the joint, ligaments, or tendons, which typically heal after a good night's sleep, would begin to accumulate in a person who did not sleep well, resulting in increased joint pain.

Smoking also diminishes the body's ability to build collagen. That is why smokers get facial wrinkles at a younger age than non-smokers. If someone was a smoker at the time he or she suffered an injury to a joint, that person's ability to make new, strong collagen fibers during the critical healing period might be compromised. Even if the person quit smoking later, the injured area would stay in an unhealed state because the stimulation for healing had already passed.

Another reason that has been suggested for incomplete healing are the use of anti-inflammatory medications immediately after an injury.[18] Inflammation is a necessary component of soft tissue healing and the use of anti-inflammatory medication for sports injuries has been questioned and remains controversial.[19] (See Chapter 9.)

Finally, if there have been too many accumulated injuries on top of each other, the joint becomes so weakened that healing is difficult.

How Does Prolotherapy Address This Problem?

Prolotherapy activates the body's healing response and stimulates growth factors in painful areas by creating a local, directed irritation to the joint area. Prolotherapy is the "stimulus" that starts the healing response, raising growth factor levels and increasing growth factor effectiveness to promote tissue repair or growth at the site of injury.[20] You could say Prolotherapy "tricks" the body into beginning a new healing cycle for injuries that have stopped healing on their own. Prolotherapy creates an irritation, sometimes called a "sterile inflammation," at the weak and painful areas. The body perceives this irritation as an injury it needs to heal and then gets busy doing what it was programmed to do—it heals that tissue!

Once ligaments and tendons are strong again, muscle spasm (which occurred as a result of the joint's instability) often resolves. And, though the osteoarthritis that has developed does not go away, a remarkable thing has been observed in many people with osteoarthritis after Prolotherapy—the *pain* reduces or goes away![21]

WHAT ARE OTHER NAMES FOR PROLOTHERAPY?

Prolotherapy is also known as "regenerative injection therapy" ("RIT"), "reconstructive therapy," "growth factor stimulation injection," or "non-surgical tendon, ligament, and joint reconstruction."[22] "Sclerotherapy" is an older, inaccurate term for Prolotherapy, based on the original theory that scar formation was how this treatment worked to make joints stronger. However, biopsy studies have not demonstrated scar formation with materials and concentrations currently in use.[23] Rather, studies have shown a proliferation of new, normal, thicker, and stronger connective tissue after Prolotherapy.[24]

SUMMARY

Most chronic musculoskeletal pain is caused by injured ligaments and tendons that have not completely healed. Prolotherapy stimulates the body to heal, strengthen, and rebuild weakened ligaments, tendons, and joints— even years after the initial injury—thereby greatly reducing or eliminating pain.

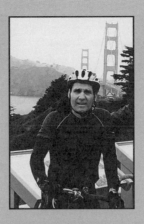

A College Instructor

I have always been a very active, athletic individual, running marathons and doing triathlons well into my 50s. About a year ago, I started to experience extreme pain in my right knee. The two orthopedic surgeons I consulted wanted to replace the knee, telling me I had degenerative arthritis and virtually no cartilage left. One of them shot me up with "Syn-visc," but this did not solve the problem. I kept looking and found out about Prolotherapy.

Prior to my Prolotherapy treatments, I could not walk up or down stairs, bend my knee past 90 degrees, or stand in front of my students for more than 20 minutes without extreme pain. My knee would constantly "snap, crackle, and pop." I ride a motorcycle and literally could not rest my right knee against the fuel tank, as the minimal vibration would cause extreme pain. My life had become grossly altered by this condition.

I was very skeptical about Prolotherapy, to be sure, but was willing to try anything that would allow me to avoid the scalpel or place artificial parts in my body. After just four Prolotherapy treatments, I was biking, swimming, and doing yoga with a freedom from pain I had not experienced in nearly two years. Just two days prior to my fifth appointment, I completed a 73-mile bike ride around Lake Tahoe, which involved a great deal of climbing. I completed the ride in just over four hours with no pain whatsoever.

I teach four 80-minute classes every other day and three classes on the alternate days, and I am on my feet for all or nearly all of that time. I no longer have to sit every 20 minutes to alleviate the pain. It's great to be able to stand in front of my students for an entire class—in fact several classes—without pain! I swim 1,500 to 2,000 yards three days a week, pain free. I bike an average of 100 miles a week, pain free, and was able to bike through Europe last summer. I do yoga, dance, hike, and walk with no pain. And there's only one explanation for this incredible turn of events: Prolotherapy works!

Joseph Spair
College Instructor

CHAPTER 4

The Medical Evidence

Many world-renowned medical centers are taking note of Prolotherapy's effectiveness. In the April 2005 issue of the Mayo Clinic Health Letter, the authors write: "In the case of chronic ligament or tendon pain that hasn't responded to more conservative treatments such as prescribed exercise and physical therapy, Prolotherapy may be helpful."[1]

Lloyd Saberski, M.D., former Medical Director of Yale University School of Medicine Center for Pain Management, writes:

> "Prolotherapy is the only methodology I have ever utilized with both limited risk yet potential for significant benefit....I routinely utilize Prolotherapy for management of mechanical low back pain and various sports-related injuries."[2]

Prolotherapy has also made its way into the sports world.[3] In a 2000 issue of *The Physician and Sportsmedicine,* the article starts:

> "Prolotherapy, considered an alternative therapy, is quietly establishing itself in mainstream medicine because of its almost irresistible draw for both physicians and patients: nonsurgical treatment for musculoskeletal conditions."

The article indicates that at that time as many as 450,000 Americans had undergone Prolotherapy and that some of the patients reporting benefits from Prolotherapy were physicians themselves.[4]

WHAT IS THE MEDICAL EVIDENCE?

Over the years since the 1930s, a long list of medical studies, reports, books, papers, and other medical literature have demonstrated the effectiveness of Prolotherapy for musculoskeletal complaints, including double-blind studies. See *APPENDIX: Prolotherapy Studies, Research Articles, and Books* for a comprehensive list of these references.

In fact, research confirms that Prolotherapy stimulates the production of growth factors that help to repair sites of injury.[5] Studies show that ligaments and tendons treated with Prolotherapy increase in strength, stability, and texture—even above normal.[6,7] Especially important in the medical world are "double-blind studies." *Double-blind* means that neither the participants nor the doctors and staff know which patients have the "real" solution or medication and which have the "placebo," thus eliminating bias and increasing accuracy of results. Such studies show Prolotherapy to be a safe and effective treatment.[8,9]

Certain studies are noteworthy. One double-blind study assessed normal rabbit tendons after Prolotherapy injections. The results were that Prolotherapy "significantly increased the mass of the ligament and strength of the [bone-ligament] junction."[10] Microscopic analysis confirmed a statistically significant increase in the collagen fibril diameters of the experimental ligament.[11] A similar animal study showed increases in the number of cells, vascular (blood) supply, and deposition of new collagen after injections.[12] Similarly, biopsies of human tissue after a series of Prolotherapy injections showed an increase in average fiber diameter from 0.55 micrometers to 0.88 micrometers, a 60 percent increase![13]

In 2001, the Florida Academy of Pain Medicine thoroughly reviewed the medical literature relating to Regenerative Injection Therapy (another name for Prolotherapy). The Academy analyzed all available reports and studies from 1937 to 2000, evaluating every reported result and including more than 530,000 patient results. Improvement in terms of return to work and previous functional/occupational activities was reported in a high percentage of patients. The procedure's safety was also evaluated and found to be low risk. The Florida Academy concluded that this treatment is "a valuable method of treatment for correctly diagnosed chronic painful conditions of the locomotive systems."[14]

The American Association of Orthopedic Medicine published its position paper specifically regarding Prolotherapy for low back pain. This paper reviewed the basic science models and reviewed the medical literature. The Association concluded that "Prolotherapy is a safe, efficacious therapy for the treatment of selected cases of low back pain and other chronic myofascial pain syndromes."[15]

A 2004 Canadian study of 177 patients treated with Prolotherapy followed their progress for up to two years. The doctors concluded that 91 percent of patients receiving Prolotherapy had reduced pain, 84 percent had improvement in their ability to work, and 85 percent could perform self-care more easily. Also of note: Of patients undergoing treatments, there were no reported complications.[16]

OTHER EVIDENCE

Prolotherapy courses are given through the University of Wisconsin School of Medicine Continuing Medical Education Department and through the American Academy of Osteopathy at the University of New England School of Osteopathic Medicine, among other places, where evidence-based medicine is important. These courses grant Continuing Medical Education (CME) credits to physicians, significant in that CME credits must be approved by our national medical associations—the American Medical Association (AMA) and the American Osteopathic Association (AOA)—in order for their doctors (M.D. or D.O.) to earn CME credits at these courses. The AMA and AOA only grant CMEs for courses that satisfy certain criteria, and a physician must earn a certain number of CME credits each year to maintain a license to practice medicine.

Long-Term Results

Long-term results for Prolotherapy have been informally reported and accountings of patient success rates tracked. Dr. George S. Hackett, one of the procedure's pioneers in the 1950s, reported an 82 percent cure rate at 12 years after Prolotherapy treatments on 1,800 patients.[17] Dr. Gustav Hemwall learned Prolotherapy from Dr. Hackett in the 1950s and then went on to treat over 10,000 patients. Dr. Hemwall studied the progress of these patients over the years. In 1974 he presented his findings to the Prolotherapy Association, reporting that out of 1,871 patients who completed Prolotherapy treatments, 75.5 percent reported complete recovery and cure, 24.3 percent reported general improvement, 0.2 percent showed no improvement, with only 9 percent of patients unable to be located. The net result of Dr. Hemwall's study was that 99 percent of surveyed patients who completed treatment found some relief from their chronic pain.[18]

While further research is still ongoing, it is clear from the dozens of studies and thousands of patient successes over the years that Prolotherapy is a highly effective treatment for chronic musculoskeletal pain.

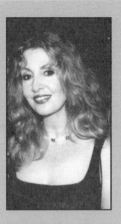

A Ballerina

I would like to tell you my story. I am an ex-professional ballet dancer and now a ballet teacher. As such, I have experienced many injuries over the years, mainly to the joints. I didn't have surgery, luckily, but over time I have had increasing immobility and pain. In the last year I started to get shoulder pain to such a degree that I could barely lift my arm. Even very small movements would cause excruciating pain so that I became almost incapacitated.

When I saw Dr. Alderman about it, even she expressed skepticism as to whether Prolotherapy could help. She told me I might have to have surgery. Well, needless to say, I didn't want to go through surgery, but given the circumstances, I decided to brave the needle (you see, I have a fear of needles) and get the Prolotherapy.

I couldn't believe it! The treatment was easier than I thought, and immediately after the injections I had more range of movement…. Already….We were both very happy with the result. As the days went on, my mobility and pain improved. After the third treatment, I felt a greater improvement to the point of almost no pain at all. Then, after the fourth treatment, I had no more pain and almost total mobility in my shoulder. Now, mind you, the pain had been unbearable….I am back to normal functioning now, after only four Prolotherapy treatments and osteopathic manipulation to help recover my shoulder range of motion after the pain improved.

I urge anyone with any kind of joint pain to find out about Prolotherapy. It WORKS!

Kathy Moore
Former Professional Ballerina
Director, The Moore Method Exercise
www.themooremethod.com

CHAPTER 5

How Prolotherapy Is Done

Prolotherapy is done in a doctor's office. The procedure involves the use of a very slender needle to inject an irritating solution to painful joint areas in order to reactivate a healing response. Injections occur at sites where a ligament or tendon attaches to bone, known as the "fibro-osseous junction" (*fibro* meaning "fibrous tissue," such as ligament or tendon, and *osseous* meaning "bone"). It is at this junction that new tissue grows; therefore, tissue repair and proliferation (regeneration or growth) can be stimulated here.

The first thing to expect when being evaluated by a doctor for Prolotherapy treatment is that he or she will take a history of the problem. The goal is to find out as much as possible about when the pain started, how it started, any prior trauma, the pain's location, what makes the pain better, what makes it worse, what has been tried already and how those treatments worked, as well as general health status. The doctor then performs a musculoskeletal physical exam, followed by a diagnosis of where he or she believes the pain is coming from. While often pain stems from an injury at the site where the pain is felt, this is not always the case. The body has a tendency toward "referred" pain, where the pain is actually coming from a remote site and travels along a referral pathway. Medicine has many examples of referred pain—for instance, tooth pain that is actually stemming from an ear infection, or a heart attack where the pain is felt in the left arm or jaw. Pain referral patterns also exist for the spine.

As you can see from the pain referral patterns demonstrated in the charts on the pages that follow, a ligament or tendon problem in the upper neck can refer pain into the head, causing headaches. Similarly, a low back problem can cause pain down the leg, a condition commonly referred to as "sciatica." And while referred pain is quite an interesting and lengthy subject, the important thing to understand here is that the pain is sometimes stemming from another site. In either case, the Prolotherapist does an evaluation to determine where the weakened ligament or tendon is—where he or she believes the pain is coming from—and then verifies that the area is appropriate for treatment.

To find the problem site, the doctor looks for tender spots and a reaction known as the "jump sign." Typically, when the doctor presses on the correct spot, the patient jumps. Sometimes, however, a person is so accustomed to his or her pain, is taking medication that covers up the pain, or has such a high tolerance for pain that these tender spots are obscured and the

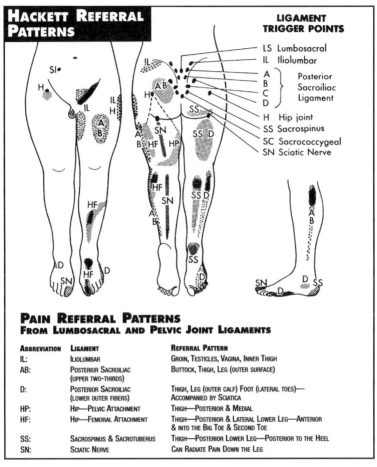

FIGURE 5-1: Ligament Referral Pain Patterns Lumbosacral Region
Reproduced by permission from Ross A. Hauser and Marion A. Hauser, *Prolo Your Pain Away!* (Oak Park, IL: Beulah Land Press, 2004), 24.

doctor fails to get a dramatic jump sign. Taking this into account and using all available information, the doctor determines if the problem is treatable and, if so, the appropriate sites to inject.

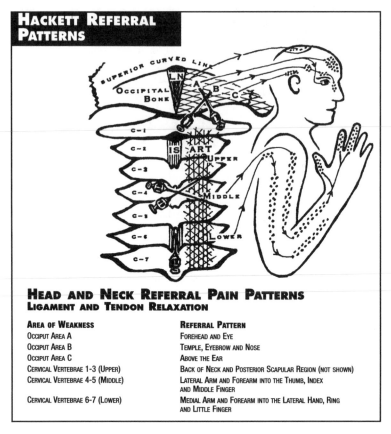

HACKETT REFERRAL PATTERNS

HEAD AND NECK REFERRAL PAIN PATTERNS
LIGAMENT AND TENDON RELAXATION

AREA OF WEAKNESS	REFERRAL PATTERN
OCCIPUT AREA A	FOREHEAD AND EYE
OCCIPUT AREA B	TEMPLE, EYEBROW AND NOSE
OCCIPUT AREA C	ABOVE THE EAR
CERVICAL VERTEBRAE 1-3 (UPPER)	BACK OF NECK AND POSTERIOR SCAPULAR REGION (NOT SHOWN)
CERVICAL VERTEBRAE 4-5 (MIDDLE)	LATERAL ARM AND FOREARM INTO THE THUMB, INDEX AND MIDDLE FINGER
CERVICAL VERTEBRAE 6-7 (LOWER)	MEDIAL ARM AND FOREARM INTO THE LATERAL HAND, RING AND LITTLE FINGER

FIGURE 5-2: **Head and Neck Ligament Referral Pain Patterns**
Reproduced by permission from Ross A. Hauser and Marion A. Hauser, *Prolo Your Pain Away!* (Oak Park, IL: Beulah Land Press, 2004), 25.

It is also important that the patient does not have any underlying health conditions that would prevent healing and is not taking any medications that would interfere with healing or Prolotherapy. The doctor will go over his or her conclusions with the patient. If both agree about the procedure, including the possible risks, a treatment is scheduled. Sometimes, if the patient is ready and time has been scheduled, treatments are done on the same day as the consultation. Sometimes the patient comes back at a later time for treatment.

The immediate reaction to treatment is different for everyone. The next-day average response is a mild to moderate stiffness and soreness at the injection sites. This usually lasts a day or two; however, for some people it can last several days. In rare cases, after-treatment pain can last longer than this. Other individuals experience immediate pain relief, which also can last for several days to weeks. Over the weeks following the Prolotherapy treatment, blood flow to the area increases, bringing nutrients, growth factors, and immune cells to the area to rebuild the injured collagen.[1]

The timeframe between visits varies with the particular problem and the doctor's protocol; however, I generally recommend a follow-up visit in three to four weeks, the idea being to simulate a normal healing time. Some individuals heal very fast and treatment can be more aggressive, for instance with athletes. In other cases, visits are more spread out. The total number of treatments will also vary, but the usual course for most areas of the body is four to six treatments, with some people requiring fewer and some requiring more.

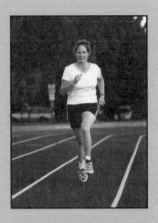

An Active Teacher

I am so excited about my full recovery. After four Prolotherapy treatments on my left hip and back, I have finally worked my way back to the pre-injury condition in that I am able to play tennis and run without any pain! I am so excited! I have been able to run the track again and do 100-yard sprints, which I could not do two years ago without falling on my face! In fact, I ran the bleacher steps at our college 12 times last night and feel no pain today at all! When I played tennis this week, I rejoiced because I no longer have to guard the way I turn and slide to get to the ball! I can concentrate on getting to the ball instead of guarding against pain!

I just recommended Prolotherapy to yet another friend who is suffering from myofacial pain and hope it will be able to help her. In fact, I have recommended it to many of my students and clients. I hope they have followed through so as to obtain the benefit of complete healing that I have! I am looking forward to backpacking with NO PAIN this summer thanks to Prolotherapy!

Diana (Shipman) Hamar
Teacher

CHAPTER 6

Why Don't More Doctors Know about Prolotherapy?

At the First Annual Injection Prolotherapy Conference, which took place in Thebes, Illinois, one of the physician attendees quite abruptly asked Dr. Gustav Hemwall, the world's most experienced Prolotherapist living at that time: "Dr. Hemwall, if Prolotherapy is so great, why don't more doctors know about it?" Dr. Hemwall paused a moment, then calmly and accurately answered, "Because it's too simple." The brash young doctor asking the question was me.

Now I am the one being asked that question. Many patients inquire, "If Prolotherapy is so good, why doesn't my doctor know about it?" The truth is that more and more doctors are finding out about Prolotherapy; however, many doctors simply have never been taught what it is or how it works. Because Prolotherapy is not taught in medical school and training must be sought out after graduation, the only way a doctor usually discovers it is "through the grapevine." Seriously. Word of mouth—hearing about other doctors who do it or about patients who have had success with it—has traditionally been the only avenue for a doctor to learn that a treatment such as Prolotherapy exists. However, the increasing number of articles being written and books being published, and even news blurbs showing up on national television and the Internet, have helped to bring Prolotherapy into public awareness. Also a few medical schools and residency programs now introduce the subject.

The first layperson's book on Prolotherapy, *Pain, Pain Go Away*,[1] was written in the late 1980s by William Faber, D.O., of the Milwaukee Pain Clinic, with co-writer William Morton, D.P.M. This was the first popular book to let the general public know such a treatment existed. In the 1990s, Ross Hauser, M.D., started writing his wonderful books on the subject. However, the real explosion of information on Prolotherapy began in this decade, with the increased use of the Internet.

In 1997, when I first created my website, **www.prolotherapy.com**, there were no other easily findable websites dedicated to Prolotherapy. That year I had only **one** patient, Bob, come to see me after doing an Internet search. Bob was a golfer with low back pain and golfer's elbow (tendonitis). He was a great guy and a wonderful patient. As I usually do with my patients, I asked Bob how he found out about Prolotherapy. He answered, "The Internet." I was stunned. I said, "Really? You use the Internet?" Remember, this was 1997, when not many people used the Internet as they do today.

I thought it was fantastic that someone actually discovered Prolotherapy that way. I knew then that the Internet was the wave of the future.

Now I see hundreds of patients each year who come in from the Web. In addition to my site, many other excellent websites address Prolotherapy, including **www.getprolo. com,** which lists doctors practicing Prolotherapy throughout the U.S. and also provides information, articles, and a free weekly email newsletter about Prolotherapy.

Dr. Hauser's book *Prolo Your Sports Injuries Away!,* for which I had the honor of writing a chapter, had many outstanding contributing authors including Lloyd Saberski, M.D., former medical director of the Yale University School of Medicine Center for Pain Management, who uses Prolotherapy in his practice. Dr. Saberski appropriately sums it up: "Prolotherapy is a secret that needs to be discovered."[2]

So times have changed. That's one thing. In addition, patients more frequently demand alternatives to drug and surgical treatments. In fact, in August 2007, *The New York Times*, one of the most widely read and respected newspapers in the world, published an article about Prolotherapy in its Personal Health section. The article states: "Since prolotherapy is a nonsurgical technique, patients who are now facing surgery because all else has failed might consider trying it before having an operation. Unlike many drugs and surgery, prolotherapy has minimal side effects when performed by an experienced practitioner..."[3]

The good news is that, although there is still a long way
to go, the word about Prolotherapy is finally getting out.

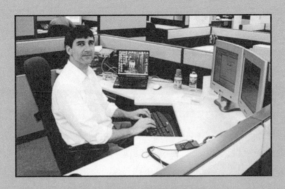

A Computer Wiz

Around the age of 20, I learned that my right leg was almost two inches longer than my left. Over the next several years I grew to have intense, agonizing back and neck pain due to my body being uneven. I eventually had surgery to shorten my right leg to make my body even. Yet, 10 years after surgery, I still lived with much back and neck pain.

For years I tried many different treatments and doctors to alleviate the pain, such as orthopedic physicians, chiropractors, physical therapists, ultrasound, massage therapy, rolfing, acupuncture, acupressure (which gave some relief), electromedical therapy (microcurrent stimulation), herbs, vitamins, and probably others that I don't recall. Thousands of dollars later I was still in pain, frustrated, out of ideas, and now very skeptical of the medical community.

Someone suggested Prolotherapy to me. I decided to research it thoroughly before possibly wasting more time, money, and energy. The concept and logic made complete sense to me. It seemed almost too simple. I was ready to try it but the skeptic inside me realized I might have another round of failures. Thankfully, I would be wrong.

My first Prolotherapy visit left my back feeling better and stronger. It was not popping out of alignment as much. I was pleasantly surprised to find something that worked—and worked fast. For my second visit, I had work done on both my back and neck. They were both getting stronger and more stable. I found it easier to focus again, which did wonders for my confidence in all social functions, especially at work.

After several visits, my back and neck are now feeling their best in 20 years! Due to that terrific success, I also had work done on my right knee and left hip, with fantastic improvements in both. I am amazed, astounded, and grateful for how good I feel today. Prolotherapy has dramatically improved my quality of life! I feel like a kid again! I often tell others who are in pain about Prolotherapy.

Jeff Confenti
Computer Engineer

CHAPTER 7

Who Is a Candidate for Prolotherapy?

One of the original medical textbooks published on Prolotherapy in the 1950s lists the following criteria as those necessary for someone to be considered a good candidate for Prolotherapy treatment:

1. Appropriate medical problem

2. Desire for recovery

3. No underlying medical conditions that would significantly interfere with healing

4. Ability and willingness to follow instructions

5. Willingness to report progress

6. Willingness to receive painful injections in an effort to recover from injury.[1]

The criteria are the same today. The problem must be an appropriate musculoskeletal one, and there needs to be a sincere desire in the patient to get well. In truth, knowing that the treatment involves injections, by the time a patient makes it to my office he or she more than likely earnestly desires recovery. In addition, there mustn't be any known illness that could prevent or interfere with healing, and there must be a willingness to follow instructions and receive the injections themselves.

It is also important that the patient not be taking medications that could interfere with the treatment, such as anti-inflammatories. Since Prolotherapy works by stimulating inflammation to produce healing, taking anti-inflammatories is counterproductive. Therefore, the patient must be willing—and able—to stop taking these medications for the duration of the Prolotherapy treatment course.

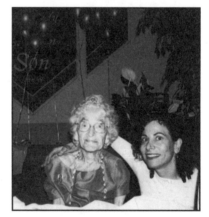

With Mary Faye at her 100th birthday party! (My birthday too!)

Age, however, is not a factor, nor does it matter how long the person has been in pain or how long ago he or she became injured, providing the person is generally in good health. Therefore, whether the injury occurred 50 years ago or 5 months ago, the person is still a candidate for treatment—again, as long as general health is good. My oldest patient, Mary Faye LaBelle, was a healthy 100 years old. Yes, 100! She received several Prolotherapy treatments and did very well. As it turned out, Mary Faye and I shared the same birthday (except for the birth year, of course!). I attended her 100th birthday party, given by her loving family.

My youngest patient was seven. Usually with children, the "willingness to undergo injection treatment" piece of the criteria is missing. This particular seven-year-old was an exception. She replied to my question, "How do you feel about shots?" with a sincere, "I just want to get better and play tennis again." And so I accepted her for treatment and she did very well, only needing a couple of treatments. I have treated many teens, usually with sports-related injuries, such as from baseball, soccer, or skateboarding. These types of patients respond well to Prolotherapy, heal well, and generally require only a few treatments.

An example of this is my patient, Shawn. He was 14 at the time I saw him, accompanied by his parents, and reported a two-year history of debilitating knee pain. He had been diagnosed with Osgood-Schlatter disease, a malady that affects many active teens. Because of the ongoing progression of his knee pain, he had given up all sports, yet his pain persisted. When I saw him, he told me, "I can't jump, I can't play any kind of sports whatsoever," then continued, "it even takes a lot of effort to walk." His parents concurred that it had been a rough couple of years. They had been told that there was no treatment for Osgood-Schlatter except anti-inflammatory medication, which would cover up the pain but not resolve it. After four Prolotherapy treatments, Shawn reported, "I can do anything now that I want to. I can run, jump, swim, play sports, go up and down stairs, and walk with no problems!" That was a few years ago, and on a recent follow-up phone call Shawn reported that the problem had never returned and that he had been able to get back to an active and athletic life.

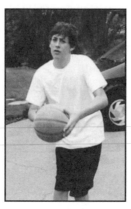

Shawn Ingallina, age 14—active again!

If you qualify, based on the above criteria, but are still not sure if you are an appropriate candidate for treatment, here are a few more questions to ask yourself. If you answer "yes" to many of them, Prolotherapy might be right for you.

1. Have you had joint pain or weakness for longer than six weeks?

2. Have you been advised to take aspirin or another anti-inflammatory medication for your pain, such as Motrin, Advil, or Aleve,

or a steroid such as cortisone for a joint, ligament, or tendon problem?

3. Have you been told you have osteoarthritis, degenerative joint disease, torn cartilage, or a bulging disc or other disc problem? Have you been told you have a chronic tendonitis?

4. Have you been told you have ligament or tendon instability, sprain-strain, or a partial tear?

5. Have you had arthroscopic surgery, orthopedic surgery, or neurosurgery and yet still experience pain?

6. Do your joints click, grind, snap, or pop?

7. Do you have a joint that buckles or slips out of place?

8. Do you need to change positions of a joint every 30 minutes (or less)?

9. Do you have a joint that swells after use?

10. In general, is your problem worse after activity or exercise (except swimming) and better at rest?

11. Does a splint or brace help the joint?

12. Does manipulation or physical therapy help, but only give temporary relief?

13. Would you prefer not to have surgery?

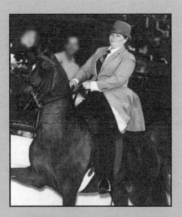

A Horse Lover and
Mary Kay Consultant

In 2005, after and MRI, I was diagnosed with osteoarthritis and three herniated discs in my neck. I was suffering with constant pain in my neck, arms, forearms, and hands and neck stiffness that would wake me up from sleeping. It got so bad that I was unable to ride my horse without experiencing terrible pain. I was told that neck fusion was the treatment, but even that wasn't recommended because of the disruption it would cause to the neck above and below the fused areas. I tried physical therapy, traction, electrical muscle stimulation, and anti-inflammatory medication; however, my pain persisted.

After Prolotherapy, I feel like a new person. I have absolutely no neck or arm pain now, and my strength has returned. I have been able to return to working out and riding my horse again, without pain, and I enjoy exercise now instead of dreading it! I have my life back!

Dawn Derenski
Mary Kay Consultant

CHAPTER 8

MRIs Can Be Misleading in Diagnosing Musculoskeletal Pain

Very often I have patients come in telling me, "Doctor, I have a ruptured disc. That's why I have this back pain," or, "I have a torn meniscus. That's why my knee hurts," or some other reason for their pain based on the results of a study known as an MRI (magnetic resonance imaging). As it turns out, however, MRIs are unreliable in correctly diagnosing musculoskeletal pain.

The simple truth is that the changes that show up in an MRI or x-ray may not be the source of a person's pain. For example, an MRI may reveal a disc bulge or other abnormality. Sure, that bulge or other abnormality is there—it does exist—but there is no way to tell how long the abnormality on the film has been there unless someone has taken regular MRIs of an area, which is rare in a healthy person. So, someone could have had this abnormal film 10 years before, at a time when he or she had no pain. Therefore, one cannot assume that a problem on an MRI is automatically the cause of the person's pain. If every irregularity that showed up in an MRI were the true cause of a person's pain, every surgery based on an MRI would result in a cure. But this doesn't always happen. MRIs have to be correlated clinically to what is going on in the individual.

Many studies have documented that abnormal MRI findings exist in large groups of pain-free individuals.[1,2,3,4,5,6,7] A study published in the *New England Journal of Medicine* showed that out of 98 **pain-free** people, 64 percent had abnormal back scans.[8] These were people with **no** pain! Additional studies have shown abnormal neck MRI scans in asymptomatic (pain-free) subjects.[9,10,11] And finding non-painful changes in knee joints during surgery is not uncommon.[12,13] One study looked at the value of MRIs in the treatment of knee injuries and concluded:

"Overall, magnetic resonance imaging diagnoses added little guidance to patient management and at times provided spurious [false] information."[14]

In the shoulder, imaging studies have discovered partial thickness and full thickness tears of the rotator cuff and other shoulder abnormalities in groups of people with **no** pain or symptoms.[15,16,17,18] A 2002 study of professional baseball pitchers concluded: **"The mere presence of signal [MRI] changes or abnormalities does not indicate pathologic symptomatic findings."**[19]

Therefore, to accurately diagnose the cause of a patient's pain, the doctor must begin by understanding the problem's history. Cyriax, one of the fathers of orthopedic medicine, said, "A doctor who doesn't have a diagnosis after the history will hardly get one after the physical examination." An imaging study should not replace a diagnosis based on history, symptom progression, and physical exam. Understanding what happened prior to the problem's onset, and not just relying on an MRI or x-ray, is very important.

On the other end of the spectrum, with musculoskeletal pain there is often a lack of conclusive objective physical signs—meaning CAT scans (computerized tomography, a sophisticated type of x-ray) or MRIs are negative or inconclusive, blood tests are normal, and x-rays show minimal or unrelated problems. Yet the pain is real; there *is* a problem. So the fact that something did or did not show up on a film may not accurately reflect the reason for a person's pain. I have patients with absolutely normal MRIs who are in chronic pain.

ABNORMAL MRIs Do Not Always Mean Surgery Is Needed!

Does an abnormal MRI now mean a person will need surgery later? A 2003 study published in the *American Journal of Sports Medicine* looked at shoulder MRIs of elite overhead athletes (those who perform repetitive "overhead" activity, such as serving and smashing in tennis, freestyle or butterfly swimming, bowling in cricket, javelin or baseball throwing, and above-shoulder weight-training exercises).[20] These athletes are more likely to suffer injury to their shoulders because of continual and repetitive use. At the study's start, **none** of the athletes had any shoulder pain or problems. Yet, on MRI **40 percent** showed partial or full thickness tears of the rotator cuff, and **20 percent** showed other abnormalities! After five years, however, **none** of the athletes interviewed had any complaints or had needed any evaluation or treatment for shoulder-related problems during the five previous years. The study's authors concluded that **"MRIs alone should not be used as a basis for operative intervention ...."**[21]

Evidence of this is reflected in a double-blind study done in July 2002, published in the *New England Journal of Medicine*, which followed two groups of patients with x-rays or MRIs showing osteoarthritis of the knee. One group received a "placebo" arthroscopic procedure, while the other received the actual treatment. After two years, this study concluded that outcomes with the actual procedure were no better than those with the placebo.[22]

It is important to remember that even in this high-tech age, radiographic tests for soft tissue injuries may not be truly diagnostic one way or the other and, therefore, should not be used alone for diagnosis. MRIs can be useful in certain circumstances but must always be correlated to the individual and his or her symptoms, and should not replace the information provided by the problem's medical history and a good musculoskeletal exam.[23]

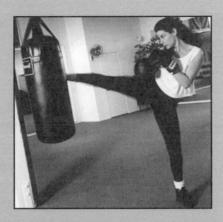

A Kickboxer and Personal Trainer

At age 23, I began studying Taekwondo for self-defense. I quickly developed a love for the martial arts and began training with a passion. Unfortunately, after a few months I injured my right knee while sparring. I didn't know it at the time, but I had injured my anterior cruciate ligament (ACL). I eventually had surgery. I was competing in Olympic Taekwondo sparring and wanted to try to compete at the 2000 Olympic trials. I was able to compete, but my performance suffered.

For several months my knee felt fine, and then the pain on the inside of the knee returned. At the same time, my low back "went out" without any warning, causing painful muscle spasms. An MRI was ordered for my right knee and revealed further damage to my medial meniscus with probable damage to my articular cartilage.

The doctor's recommendation for my knee was grim—another surgery, a high tibial osteotomy. This very serious surgery involves cutting through most of the tibia, changing the angle of the bone, and plating it to create more space on the inside of the knee. The surgery permanently deforms the leg. I was devastated and sought a second opinion. The second doctor was more conservative and recommended arthroscopic surgery to access the damage. I decided to go forward with the scope, which confirmed the earlier diagnosis of damage to my articular cartilage.

Holes were drilled in the areas of exposed bone to facilitate the regrowth of makeshift cartilage. The surgery provided only temporary relief. I was told to take pain and anti-inflammatory medication.

A few months later, I found myself searching the Internet for alternative therapies for my knee pain. I stumbled upon Prolotherapy. At my first appointment, I had my knee treated and was very excited with the results. The almost-constant pain on the inside of my knee was greatly reduced. I was able to return to most of my physical activities without pain, including martial arts. At my second visit, I was in the middle of a back flare-up and decided to try Prolo on my low back. I was very impressed with the immediate pain relief I experienced. Over the last nine months, I have received six treatments on my knee and three on my back with great success. My back rarely flares up and when it does, the pain is minimal. My knee has also continued to improve, allowing me to teach my fitness classes without pain. I have also had a couple of treatments on my neck and shoulder, for old injuries that have recently resurfaced. My neck pain has disappeared.

At age 33, I have learned a great deal about how the body heals (or doesn't heal) since my first injury 10 years ago. I now know that surgery and anti-inflammatory drugs are not the answer for most soft tissue injuries. Instead of working against the body's natural ability to heal, Prolo works in concert with the healing process. I am now committed to resting and aiding the body in healing itself. I am also committed to spreading the word about the benefits of Prolotherapy.

Jennifer Freitas
Personal Trainer

CHAPTER 9

Think Twice Before
Taking Pain Medication

In October 2003 Rush Limbaugh, a well-known syndicated radio talk show host, shocked many people when he admitted his addiction to narcotic prescription pain medication. What began as a temporary solution for pain turned into a long-term obsession that interfered with his daily life and, of course, never permanently resolved the cause of his pain.

The short-term use of pain medication is at times warranted, but, unfortunately, long-term use of narcotics can too often develop into a downward spiral. Evidence suggests that narcotics, as well as anti-inflammatory medications—which are frequently used to ease musculoskeletal pain—reduce the body's ability to heal the very injuries they are being taken for and have potentially serious side effects.[1,2,3]

Narcotics Can Lower Immune Function and Impair Healing

The term *narcotic* is actually the older name for a class of medications now called "opioid analgesics." This class includes morphine, codeine, OxyContin, and Vicodin, among others. For more than 100 years, opioids have been observed to negatively affect the immune system.[4] Researchers at the University of Minnesota state, "Overwhelming evidence suggests that opioid use affects ... immunity."[5] Italian researchers agree, noting, "Recent studies suggest that opioids can have an adverse impact on the immune system."[6] Research at Temple University School of Medicine in Philadelphia provides evidence that opioid medications do indeed prevent a type of immune cell from working to repair an injured area or from fighting off infection.[7] Interestingly, studies with both animal and human cancer cells showed that opioid medications can increase the size and spread of the cancer cells.[8,9,10,11] Clearly, opioids have the ability to negatively impact healing and should be used sparingly, short term, and only when absolutely necessary.

Anti-Inflammatory Medications Can Prevent Soft Tissue Healing and Have Side Effects

NSAIDs ("non-steroidal anti-inflammatory medications") are among the most commonly prescribed drugs in the United States, with widespread use in treating acute musculoskeletal injuries.[12,13] There are two types of NSAIDs—the original and the newer versions. The original NSAIDs include ibuprofen (brand name Motrin or Advil), naproxen (brand name Aleve), voltarin, and others. This group has the undesirable side effect of stopping the production of protective stomach mucus, which can lead to stomach injury. Newer NSAIDs include Vioxx, Celebrex, and Bextra, among others (see end of chapter for more examples). These NSAIDs were supposed to be an improvement, as they were developed to prevent the undesirable side effect of stomach injury. Unfortunately, some members of this newer class of anti-inflammatories have been shown to increase risk of heart attacks and strokes, leading to the recall of Vioxx in 2004.[14] Both groups of NSAIDs work by stopping inflammation, and both have been questioned for use in musculoskeletal injuries.[15,16]

NSAIDs are commonly prescribed for such complaints as muscle injuries, ligament sprains, tendon injuries, low back pain, and osteoarthritis. However, using NSAIDs for soft tissue and sports injuries has been questioned in recent years.[17] Studies have shown that using NSAIDs for these types of injuries may delay the healing response and slow the rate of recovery of strength in the muscle-tendon unit.[18,19,20,21]

STRIKE WHILE THE IRON IS HOT: DECREASING INFLAMMATION IS COUNTERPRODUCTIVE

Before we go any further, we need to ask ourselves, "Do we really want to stop inflammation in soft tissue injuries?" Researchers agree that inflammation is a necessary component in the healing process.[22] Blocking inflammation means decreased blood flow, resulting in less healing of musculoskeletal injuries.[23] Although given by well-meaning physicians to stop pain in the short run, in the long run there are concerns that NSAIDs may decrease healing during the early and critical healing phases after an injury.[24]

If the body is injured today, the impetus to heal is *now*. Therefore, we want to make sure that all conditions for healing are optimal. As they say, it's best to strike while the iron is hot. If we diminish inflammation during the critical healing period, the body may not mend completely. Remember from Chapter 2: Prolotherapy Basics that after the body's timeframe for initial healing has passed (four to six weeks from the time of injury), the stimulation to heal is lessened significantly (i.e., the iron has "cooled off"). The body will not try to do much healing after this point; therefore, whatever healing has occurred up until then—whether a little or a lot—is usually what the person is left with. So why slow down the process during this critical period?

Studies Show NSAIDs Reduce Healing of Ligaments

In 1997, researchers conducted a study of 364 Australian army recruits with ankle sprains. One group was given NSAIDs, while the other was not. The group given NSAIDs returned to activity sooner, probably because of decreased pain; however, the NSAIDs group also had more ankle instability and decreased range of motion, as compared with the placebo (non-medicated) group.[25]

A 2001 animal study took a look at the effects of NSAIDs on ligament healing. Fifty rats with the same knee ligament injury were divided into two groups. Half of the rats were given an NSAID; the other half, a placebo. Two weeks later, the ligaments were tested. The group given NSAIDs were found to have 32 percent weaker ligament strength than those given placebo.[26]

NSAIDs May Delay Muscle Healing

In general, muscles have a good blood supply and heal quickly. However, recent evidence shows that NSAIDs may delay healing in muscle stretch injuries. In a study of athletes with acute hamstring injuries, one group was given NSAIDs while another was given placebo. After the treatment period, when both groups were no longer being medicated, the researchers noted that pain reduction was better in the placebo (non-medicated) group than in the NSAIDs group, inferring that better overall healing had occurred without the drugs. They concluded that using NSAIDs for muscular injuries was not recommended.[27] Other researchers agree that while NSAIDs may help with symptoms and pain, there is concern that using these drugs is associated with negative effects later in the healing phase.[27]

NSAIDs MAY PREVENT BONE HEALING

Evidence also exists that using NSAIDs during the critical period after bone injury may prevent healing. A study examined 288 patients who underwent spinal fusion, an operation where two bones in the spine are fused together. The patients who took NSAIDs in the period immediately following surgery were compared to those who did not. This study determined that those patients who took the NSAIDs were five times more likely to not heal, to experience "fusion non-union" (meaning the bones didn't grow together).[29] The authors recommended that these drugs be avoided in the early healing period after surgery. Another study focused on 67 patients who had suffered a hip fracture. This study concluded that there was a marked association with failure to heal and delayed healing in patients who had taken NSAIDs.[30]

Animal studies have also raised questions about how NSAIDs affect bone healing. A study done in May 2002 divided 253 rats into four groups. Three of the groups each received a different type of NSAID, and the fourth group received no treatment or just a "water" (placebo) treatment. The researchers found that the placebo group had regular and good bone healing, while the other three groups had delayed bone healing—from one week to as much as incomplete healing after eight weeks, depending on the group.[31] The chairman of the Department of Orthopaedic Surgery at the Boston University School of Medicine calls these findings "compelling" and advises that it would be "prudent" to temporarily avoid or discontinue using NSAIDs during a period of bone healing.[32]

USING NSAIDs IN TENDONITIS IS QUESTIONABLE

Tendonitis is the term used to describe inflammation ("itis") of a tendon. However, in recent years biopsies of tissues labeled as "tendonitis" have revealed something very interesting: Tendonitis may not be an inflammatory condition after all! As will be discussed later in this book, growing evidence shows that tendonitis is actually "tendon*osis*," a condition where there is no inflammation but rather degeneration of the tendon's collagen with failure to heal.[33] Therefore, using an agent that stops inflammation where no inflammation exists and that also has the potential to delay healing is particularly questionable.

NSAIDs HAVE SIDE EFFECTS

And there's more! Using NSAIDs in general can raise blood pressure, worsening the problem in someone with already increased levels.[34] These medications can also increase dehydration in athletes and have been implicated in some case reports of kidney failure in marathoners.[35,36] Another study evaluated NSAID use in the general population and concluded that long-term use of this type of medication increases the risk of kidney failure.[37]

Complications related to gastrointestinal (stomach, intestine) side effects from using NSAIDs are responsible for approximately 100,000 hospital admissions with 16,500 deaths in the U.S. each year. In fact, gastrointestinal bleeding from NSAID use is the 15th leading cause of death in the U.S.[38]

These figures do not even include deaths that may be related to using Vioxx, a member of the newer class of NSAIDs. In a discontinued medical study, patients taking Vioxx for more than 18 months had approximately twice as many heart attacks and strokes as those not taking the drug.[39] Although the reason for these complications is not completely clear, it is believed that in addition to inhibiting the enzyme that causes inflammation, Vioxx inhibits an enzyme that protects the heart by dilating blood vessels and preventing clots.[40] Because of these findings Vioxx was pulled from the market in 2004, and some other NSAIDs in the same class are now under close scrutiny.

NSAIDS AND PROLOTHERAPY

The bottom line is that inflammation is necessary for healing[41] and is therefore an important component for effective treatment using Prolotherapy. Without inflammation, there can be no healing response and thus no new healing. Because of this, Prolotherapy patients are instructed not to take anti-inflammatory medications during their course of treatment. Patients who are on narcotic pain medication are advised to restrict usage as much as possible, so that the immune system may function optimally.

Examples of NSAIDs[42]

Over-the-Counter NSAIDs
Ibuprofen (ADVIL, MOTRIN IB)

Ketoprofen (ACTRON-, ORUDIS KT)

Naproxen sodium (ALEVE)

Prescription NSAIDs
Celecoxib (CELEBREX)

Diclofenac potassium (CATAFLAM)

Diclofenac sodium (VOLTAREN)

Etodolac (LODINE)

Fenoprofen (NALFON)

Flurbiprofen (ANSAID)

Ibuprofen (MOTRIN)

Indomethacin (INDOCIN)

Ketoprofen (ORUVAIL)

Lumiracoxib (PREXIGE)

Meclofenamate sodium (MECLOMEN)

Meloxicam (MOBIC)

Nabumetone (RELAFEN)

Naproxyn (NAPROSYN)

Oxaprozin (DAYPRO)

Piroxicam (FELDENE)

Rofecoxib (VIOXX)

Sunlindac (CLINORIL)

Tolmetin sodium (TOLECTIN)

Valdecoxib (BEXTRA)

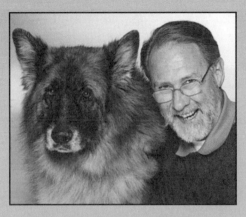

A Financial Estate Planner

In 1982 I was packing for a move from San Diego to Denver. I bent over at the waist, slightly twisting to the left, and picked up a small television set. I was at that time 40 years young and, I thought, in great shape. It felt like 440 volts hit me in my lower left back. I immediately went to a chiropractor friend of mine who adjusted me, and the injury seemed to stabilize. The relief only lasted a few days; then the pain returned.

I flew to Denver. As soon as I tried to get up in the plane I knew I had a big problem. I was taken off in a wheelchair. I started seeing chiropractors three times a day—crying in pain while lying on the table, begging, "Please help me." To no avail. As long as I was upright I was okay. If I sat down I knew it was going to take going to the floor and crawling to the wall to begin a 15-minute process of standing up straight again. There was no way I was able to stand up without assistance. The last few degrees to upright were the longest. Once upright, I was pain free.

Then I discovered Advil. I ate Advil like it was candy, finding that I could function with the pain level down to an aggravation rather than paralyzing. Over time I weaned myself off the Advil. However, after multiple chiropractors, multiple M.D.s, an MRI that showed a slight bulge in a disc—nothing more—massage therapy and on and on, I just gave up and started living with the pain, a tight hamstring, and muscle cramps in my left hamstring.

I was afraid to exercise and moved around like on eggshells. In 1996 I acquired a service dog to help me get around.

Then in 2003—after suffering for over 20 years—while searching the Internet, Googling on "pain," I came across the term *Prolotherapy*. I'd never heard of it. With more searching, I found that Dr. C. Everett Koop mentions it on his site and has had it done as a patient and recommends it.

More searching led me to the "Princess of Prolotherapy," Dr. Donna Alderman, who has a practice not 10 minutes from my home. I immediately made an appointment, and on June 24, 2003, I knew that I had finally found what I needed. The first treatment eliminated 100 percent of the pain immediately. I knew that it would come back over the next weeks, that it was a healing process and that it would take multiple treatments to eliminate the pain for good.

That evening while sharing dinner with my older sister and telling her of my experience, I started crying for the relief of ending over 20 years of pain and disability. The tears soon turned to laughter over my newfound joy of my life being reestablished. It had been a long, hard, expensive trip.

During the weeks between treatment—my body would tell me when it was time for the next session—I couldn't wait to see "Dr. Dawna" again.

On March 24, 2004, Dr. Alderman presented me with a T-shirt and "kicked me out." It had been six months since my last treatment.

Now, more than two years later, I am still enjoying the benefits of those Prolotherapy sessions. And much to my now-retired service dog's enjoyment, we actually get off the sidewalks and get out in the country for lengthy walks and play.

Bob Dillon
Financial Estate Planner

CHAPTER 10

Prolotherapy for Low Back Pain

L ow back pain affects most people at some point during their lifetime. It is the second most frequently reported illness in industrialized countries, next to the common cold.[1] In fact, it has been reported that 80 percent of the general U.S. population will at some time suffer from low back pain, and 20 percent are suffering at any given time.[2,3] In the United States it is estimated that more than 5 million people are disabled by low back pain, half of whom are permanently disabled.[4] Mechanical low back pain (meaning caused by overuse or by lifting, straining, or bending injuries) is the most common cause of work-related disability in persons under 45 years old.[5] A variety of sports activities, such as gymnastics, football, weight lifting, rowing, golf, dance, tennis, baseball, basketball, and cycling, have been linked to low back pain.[6] Nonathletes and athletes alike, however, can suffer from this common condition. Low back pain is the subject of numerous books, articles, and media reports.

Despite advanced medical technology, the number of patients suffering from back pain continues to increase.[7] Although, as you have read, it has been well documented that MRIs are not specific enough to guarantee that the detected lesions are the source of a person's pain (see Chapter 8), many surgeons base their decisions to operate primarily on the outcome of these investigations.[8] It is inevitable, then, that some of the surgeries done are not necessary and will not resolve the pain for which they are intended.

COMMON CAUSES OF LOW BACK PAIN

Most low back pain (estimated at 90 percent) is caused by overuse or straining, spraining, lifting, or bending that results in ligament sprains, muscle pulls, or disc herniations.[9] This is referred to as "mechanical low back pain." As a doctor in training, I observed that many young mothers began having low back pain just as their infants reached 30 pounds. On further questioning, I discovered that the way they were lifting their children had not changed from when the infants were only 8 pounds. But now they were lifting more than three times the weight! Correcting the biomechanics of how they lifted the children often solved the problem. However, not all cases of low back pain are so simple to solve.

Other reasons for low back pain, usually more chronic, include osteoarthritis (irritation of a joint caused by calcium deposits or spurs in the joint) and spinal stenosis, also called central canal stenosis (a condition where the spinal canal has become narrowed because of arthritis or other degenerative changes).

Low back pain can occur with a sudden trauma; however, it typically occurs over a period of time and may not be noticed by an individual until it has progressed. Low back pain can be acute (meaning it comes on suddenly, for only a short course) or chronic (meaning it tends to come on slower and lasts longer than three months). Risk factors for low back pain run the gamut and include increased age, previous episodes of low back pain, hard physical labor, posture, or activities such as lifting with straight legs and bending while carrying heavy loads that increase physical stress on the spine, mental stress, osteoporosis, and even physical inactivity.[10] While most people recover from an acute episode of back pain, some continue to have recurrent flare-ups, and some go on to develop chronic low back pain.

WHEN IS AN ACUTE PROBLEM CONSIDERED "CHRONIC"?

Opinions about this vary. For ligament sprains, one authority considers that after six weeks an injury is chronic.[11] However, most medical authorities agree that a problem such as low back pain is chronic after it has continued for more than three months.[12]

THE MRI MYTH ABOUT DISC PROBLEMS

Far too often patients with chronic low back pain attribute their pain to a herniated disc, diagnosed based on an MRI. However, as noted in Chapter 8, MRIs can be misleading in diagnosing this kind of pain. A well-respected textbook of Orthopedic Medicine states, "The results of radiographic examinations should never be given to the patient as a diagnosis."[13] This is because, as we have already learned and as medical studies have documented over and over again, what the MRI shows may not be the reason for the person's pain. In fact, though this diagnosis is frequently given to the patient as the cause of pain, it has been reported that **only 4 percent of low back pain is due to a herniated disc.**[14]

While disc problems have gotten much of the credit, ligament injury is a more important source of back pain.[15] When and why did all this attention on disc disease begin? In 1934 researchers named Mixter and Barr became popular.[16] They focused attention on the disc, giving root to a popular theory; from that time forward, "disc disease" has overshadowed ligaments' importance. Then, with the introduction of cat scanners (CT) in the 1970s, and the popularity of MRIs in the 1980s and 1990s, further attention was focused on the disc as the cause of low back pain—because discs are easily seen in these types of studies. It seems that part of our Western culture is: "If you can see it, it must be real." And, by extension, "If you don't see it, it doesn't exist."

MRIs show disc herniations; however, they do not reveal how old those herniations are. Understandably, patients—and their doctors—are eager to find the cause of their pain. An abnormality on an MRI provides them with that seemingly obvious "reason." But, as previously noted, that herniation may not be the cause of the pain. And, if the herniation is used as the only basis for a treatment plan, the person's pain may not improve.

On the other hand, ligament injury is difficult to prove by MRI or CT. Because these injuries often involve very small but painful micro-tears, they do not usually show up on those investigations unless there is a large tear or rupture, which is less common.

Even with a History of Disc Herniation, Prolotherapy Can Help Low Back Pain

In my experience, ligament injury and laxity is the primary cause of mechanical low back pain and, in many cases, can be resolved with Prolotherapy. Even if there is a history of disc herniation, or disc herniation shows up on an MRI, this only further proves that ligaments around the disc are weak and in need of treatment.

Even after someone has "recovered" from a back injury to the point that he or she is out of severe pain, where ligaments and tendons are weak there still exists a predisposition to further injury. Prolotherapy can help stabilize and strengthen the ligaments around these weakened joints and reduce or eliminate pain.

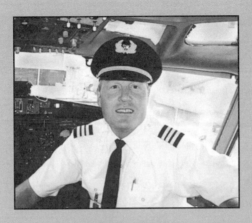

An Airline Pilot

I am a 41-year-old airline pilot and father of five who discovered Dr. Donna Alderman 19 months ago when I was in desperate need of help. My situation would have been diagnosed as "degenerative disc disease" or "failed back syndrome." I had already undergone two disc surgeries at L4/5, which had failed, but was still in pain.

During my first visit to Dr. Alderman, I explained that subsequent to my last surgery I had been up against a wall in my recovery despite a 17-month effort of faithfully doing all the right things. I have always been an athlete—basketball, surfing, bicycle racing, etc.—and despite my zealous efforts at rehab I was limping through life barely able to function. It was especially difficult performing my job as a pilot because of the pain involved in sitting.

After a thorough examination, I was thrilled when Dr. Alderman said I was a candidate for "Prolo." We began that day with the injections. Does it hurt? If you are reading this you can more than handle it, especially when you know it will bring real healing to your body.

I have now had 13 series of injections, each spaced about a month apart. This is more than most people would require due to the serious nature of my back injury. My improvement was almost immediate and has continued to build. There have been ups and downs but the lows became shallower and the highs became higher. I am so enthusiastic about Prolotherapy; hardly a week goes by that I don't tell several people about it. My wife, daughter, mom, brothers, and several friends have all succumbed to my testimony and are now fellow "Prolo-ites." I have combined these treatments with a good diet, plenty of sleep, and a steady regimen of exercises centered on lap swimming.

I recently hiked to the top of Mt. Wilson, 4,500 feet of elevation gain over seven miles, and my back felt great. I am now able to sit for extended periods of time without pain—what a difference this has made. I feel like I have been given my life back. If you are suffering from any kind of joint pain and desire real healing and strength, you must give Prolotherapy a try.

Dann Shubin
Airline Pilot

CHAPTER 11

Prolotherapy for Disc Disease

As we learned in the previous chapter, a common diagnosis for neck or back pain is "bulging disc" or "disc herniation." Because this diagnosis is so common, it deserves a chapter of its own.

During recent years the idea has become accepted by the general public that a herniated disc requires surgery, especially if the pain has not resolved after a few weeks and there is a positive MRI or CT. However common, this opinion has not been supported by the long-term studies, which show equally good or better results after conservative non-surgical treatment. Two studies found no difference between final results of surgical and non-surgical therapy after 7 and 20 years of observation.[1,2] Another study found a 92 percent return-to-work rate in a group treated conservatively, even though 60 percent had muscle weakness and 26 percent showed disc rupture on the CT scan.[3] Therefore, the presence of even large herniations and/or disc ruptures should not be taken as an absolute reason for surgery.[4,5,6] Due to the risks involved in surgery, conservative treatment should always be undertaken first. This includes Prolotherapy.

Disc Composition

To understand disc disease and what it really means, it is important to be familiar with the spine's anatomy. A disc is a circular, collagen-type tissue that sits between the bones in the spine (vertebrae). The disc acts like a cushion and shock absorber between the vertebrae to allow easier bending. The center of the disc is mainly a gelatinous, watery material called the "nucleus pulposus" (Latin for "center pulp") and is composed of a gel-like substance that has no nerve or blood supply. The outer edges are made of a ligament material called the "annulus fibrosus" (Latin for "fibrous ring") that is composed of strong ligament-like fibers that do have nerve endings, however, again, no direct blood supply. Because of this lack of blood, discs do not regenerate well when injured.

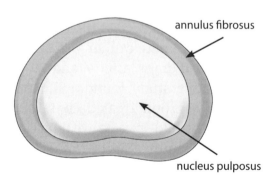

annulus fibrosus

nucleus pulposus

The center of the disc, the nucleus pulposus, is 85 percent water in a young person, but over time dehydrates and is less than 65 percent water in the elderly.[7] So, as a person ages, the discs have more tendency to lose flexibility and can be injured more easily. And, as noted, with no blood supply, discs lack the ability to regenerate and repair themselves. Once flattened, they remain so.

Disc bulge, herniation, and rupture are terms used to describe disc disease. All three are part of the same process, with bulge being the first stage, herniation next, and then rupture the most severe, signifying that fluid has leaked out of the disc through cracks around its edge. These conditions are usually diagnosed from an MRI. Though it sounds bad, and may come up on an MRI as a finding, please remember that only 4 percent of low back pain is actually due to disc disease.[8]

THE CYCLE OF A DISC HERNIATION

When a disc first herniates, it is painful—in fact, so painful that the person usually cannot walk and is literally "flat on his or her back" for several days. But, in a few days to a few weeks, the protruding disc segment slowly shrivels away.[9] In fact, with or without treatment, most disc herniations reabsorb and resolve within two to six weeks, with up to 90 percent back-to-normal activity within one month regardless of treatment.[10,11]

However, it has been estimated that 10 percent of people who suffer a disc herniation continue to have pain and go on to experience chronic back pain that includes muscle pain, spasm, and stiffness (a sign of a ligament laxity and a weak joint), sometimes with pain going down the legs. These symptoms may persist long after the disc herniation itself has shriveled away. Why does the pain persist in these people?

It is important to understand why a disc herniates. Relaxation of the spinal ligaments precedes disc herniations.[12] First, the ligaments surrounding the disc weaken, allowing the disc to herniate. Once the herniation heals, the ligament weakness remains. The joint is now even more unstable, causing continued pain. And remember, even if the herniation still shows up on an MRI, it may not be the reason for the pain.

DISCS FLATTEN OVER TIME AS A NATURAL PROCESS OF AGING

As part of the natural process of aging, discs in the neck and back become flatter over time. Certain physical activities such as bending forward, lifting heavy objects with straight knees, and even sitting for long periods of time put extra and undue strain on the discs, leading to flattening and dehydration. This, along with the decreased healing ability of the disc (remember, no blood supply), makes the disc prone to what is known as "degeneration." Disc degeneration is so common it is considered part of the normal aging process.[13]

Causes of Disc Herniations and Ruptures

For a disc to herniate, there must first be a primary ligament weakness and a deteriorating disc.[14] As discussed
above, in the natural course of aging a disc loses pliabil-
ity and is less able to withstand normal pressures. Thus,
it is more prone to having its outside edges become
cracked or torn.[15] If the pressure goes high enough, the
fluid in the disc's center can leak through these cracks
or fissures. This also leads to decreased disc height. In
addition, the ligament that holds the disc in place becomes weakened. As a result, the joint becomes even
more unstable and more likely to herniate. Simply
put, ligaments hold the disc in place, so if the ligament
weakens, the disc can more easily herniate through it.
In fact, increased pressure in the disc together with
increased ligament laxity is the perfect recipe for disc
herniation.[16,17]

While someone can suffer a disc herniation because
of sudden or severe trauma, such as lifting a heavy
box, most herniations occur over time due to repetitive
trauma—some large, some small.[18] There may not even
be a prior history of back pain, when one day a minor
event such as a cough or sneeze—or no event at all—is
enough to cause herniation of the disc material, resulting in pain.[19,20]

I have had numerous patients tell me a similar story:
"I was just lifting a plate out of the sink," or "I was just
getting out of a car," or "I was just sneezing" when suddenly they have such severe back pain it brings them to

their knees. While the innocent activity seems to be the cause, it was really just "the straw that broke the camel's back." Most people don't notice the slow process of de-generation over time and so usually don't know an area has weakened—that is, until the camel's back breaks.

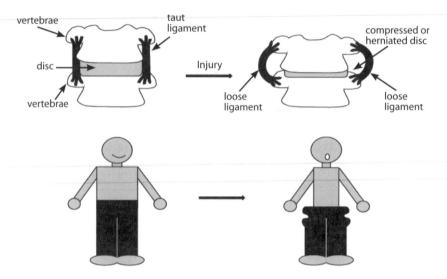

What Happens to the Ligament When the Disc Flattens

As the disc loses moisture and flattens over time, the ligament that connects the two vertebrae above and below it is now too large in comparison to the newly slimmed-down disc. Imagine someone losing six inches around his or her waist, but not tightening his or her belt....Well, you get the picture!

This situation of a flatter disc with the same (or stretched) ligament length results in more motion (instability), which causes even more strain on the disc and joint. This change in biomechanics, even with normal motion, makes the disc even more likely to flatten, leading to even more joint movement, instability, and weakness, and a dwindling cycle that, unless broken, ends up creating more pain. One problem leads to another ... and another ... and another! It's a vicious cycle. The good news is, Prolotherapy can help break it.

IS PROLOTHERAPY HELPFUL FOR SCIATICA?

Patients with a history of low back pain commonly develop sciatica, pain that runs out into the buttocks and down the legs. The term *sciatica* is often used to describe any type of pain that follows this general course. However, as mentioned previously, referral pain is common in the body. Sciatica-type pain can occur as a result of weak ligaments in the low back and sacro-iliac region along ligament referral pathways. *(See FIGURE 5-1: Ligament Referral Pain Patterns Lumbosacral Region, pg. 47)*

Just as a sprained ankle does, the low back and sacro-iliac ligaments swell when injured. Because there is not much space in the low back area, swelling can put pressure on the sciatic or other nerve roots, causing "sciatica." This is especially true when the tendons of the piriformis are irritated, because the piriformis muscle runs directly over the large sciatic nerve. Imagine what might happen if the piriformis tendon swells!

Prolotherapy has been shown to help with sciatica. A study by John Merriman compared Prolotherapy to fusion for sciatic pain. His conclusion was that 80–90

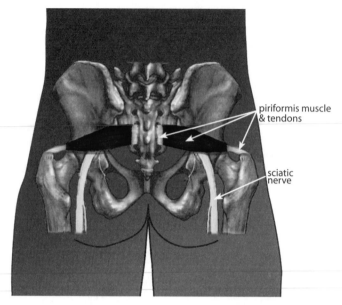

piriformis muscle
& tendons

sciatic
nerve

Piriformis Muscle over Sciatic Nerve

percent of more than 15,000 patients experienced relief from sciatica with Prolotherapy, with fewer side effects than with a fusion operation.[21]

In my experience, Prolotherapy can indeed help sciatica symptoms as long as the cause of the sciatica is not true nerve root compression or central canal stenosis (where the spinal cord is being made smaller by arthritic changes). While these conditions exist, and should be considered, the more common reasons for sciatica are soft tissue inflammation around the joint putting pressure on the nerve, causing pain. If the ligamentous or tendon damage is addressed and stimulated to heal, then the referral pain down the leg goes away. As long as there are no neurological danger signs, such as loss of feeling or function in the leg, loss of bowel or bladder function, or loss of movement, a conservative course of treatment such as Prolotherapy is reasonable.

PROLOTHERAPY CAN HELP DISC DISEASE

It is important to get a correct assessment of the reason for low back pain and to realize that only a very small percentage of disc herniations truly require surgery.[22] It is also important to understand that ligament weakness or instability predispose someone to back injury and disc herniations. Even after a disc herniation heals there may be continued pain and joint weakness, because the reason for the injury (ligament weakness) has not been resolved. There may also be muscular spasm, tightness, and pain—the body's way of trying to stabilize the area—causing further pain. Prolotherapy can help strengthen weakened tendons or ligaments, help to prevent further progression, and reduce or eliminate pain.

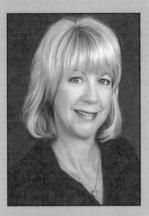

A Real Estate Agent and
Former Court Reporter

I was a court reporter for 22 years, and experienced repetitive trauma to both my elbows. Finally, I was diagnosed with chronic epicondylitis and tendonitis. I tried NSAIDs, braces, cortisone; however, my elbows continued to hurt 24/7. I experienced a constant penetrating ache and they felt bruised or like they had been slammed with a hammer.

After Prolotherapy, I have regained the use of my elbows and have more endurance. My pain is no longer constant, and I no longer have burning and tightness in my forearms. Two years after finishing my Prolotherapy treatments, I am still 95 percent improved. I am able to live life now without chronic pain. I recommend this treatment highly.

Brenda Falvi
Real Estate Agent
Orange County, California
www.brendaforhomes.com

CHAPTER 12

Prolotherapy for Chronic Tendonitis/Tendonosis, Sprains/Strains

Sprains and strains are common and can occur to any joint. A sprain is an overstretching injury to a ligament, while a strain is an overstretching injury to a tendon. For example, a sprained ankle is when the ankle's ligaments get stretched out in the wrong direction. This typically happens with a sudden twisting motion. These types of injuries are common in sports.

You will remember from previous chapters that ligaments and tendons have a poor blood supply and therefore heal slowly. In fact, it has been estimated that even under the best of circumstances, the most an injured person can hope for is 50–70 percent of pre-injury strength after a sprain.[1] Strains that do not heal can result in "tendonitis," meaning an inflammation of the tendon—a common diagnosis in sports medicine.

Tendonitis can develop in any joint in the body. Common areas for tendonitis are the elbow (for example, tennis elbow or golfer's elbow), shoulder (in the rotator cuff or biceps), and ankle (in the Achilles). However, any tendon has the potential to become inflamed and irritated, especially in sports where overuse can occur. In most cases in a healthy, non-stressed, non-smoking person, an area will heal in four to six weeks, depending on the injury's severity. However, in some cases the tendons do not heal, causing long-lasting and chronic pain. This condition is usually referred to as "chronic tendonitis."

In recent years, the term *tendonosis* ("osis" meaning diseased or abnormal condition) has been more frequently used. This refers to a condition where inflammation is no longer occurring and instead collagen breakdown is the primary problem. Some authors believe that tendonosis is more common than chronic tendonitis and that what has typically been deemed "chronic tendonitis" would more accurately be labeled "chronic tendonosis."[2,3,4] As this belief has taken root in the sports medicine community, the treatment more often recommended is one that targets stimulating collagen production rather than eliminating inflammation, which may not even be present.[5]

Studies have been done in support of this belief. One, involving biopsies of patients operated on for tendon pain and "chronic tendonitis," showed these samples *not* to have inflammation at all; in fact, the degeneration of the tendon fibers was seen with an absence of classic inflammatory cells.[6] For this reason, using anti-inflammatory medication makes even less sense. A review of the role of anti-inflammatory medication in soft tissue conditions found little evidence of effectiveness in resolving these disorders.[7] In the case of tendonosis, inflammation is absent and collagen breakdown is occurring faster than it is being rebuilt. So, what now?

Because Prolotherapy stimulates inflammation and the proliferation (i.e., growth, repair) of injured tendons and ligaments that have not healed on their own, it has been used for these conditions. Evidence shows that injecting even a low concentration of dextrose, commonly used in Prolotherapy, stimulates growth factor production to elevate within minutes to hours. With tendonosis we are trying to turn the tendon back into a tendonitis, on purpose, in order to stimulate the repair and rebuilding of collagen fibers, strengthening the joint and reducing or eliminating pain.[8,9,10,11] In my experience, chronic tendonitis and/or tendonosis as well as chronically sprained ligaments, in general, respond very well to Prolotherapy.

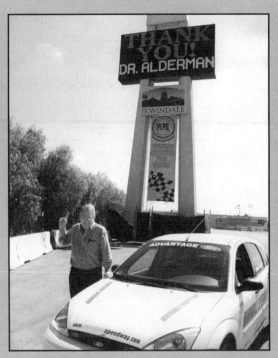

A Public Relations Executive

I found Prolotherapy while searching on the Internet for the best brand/style of a total knee replacement because I was told that was all that was left for me. After seven Prolotherapy treatments on the left, and six on the right, both of my knees are so much better. I am no longer thinking about knee replacement. There is far less pain under load, when resting in bed, better flexibility, and virtually no stiffness upon getting up after sitting at a desk or in the car for a long time, so much so that I sometimes forget that I've had "knee problems" for over 20 years. My mantra: "Yes the shots hurt. Yes, your insurance might not cover it (mine doesn't), and yes, I happily undergo the five minutes or so of discomfort because of the remarkable results that it yields."

Doug Stokes
Public Relations Executive

CHAPTER 13

Prolotherapy for Osteoarthritis

"Arthritis" is another diagnosis frequently assigned to joint pain. The word itself comes from *arthr*, meaning "joint," and *itis*, meaning "inflammation." There are several different types of arthritis, the most common being osteoarthritis (*osteo*, meaning "bone"), also known as "degenerative joint disease." As discussed earlier, osteoarthritis is diagnosed when bony spurs, calcium deposits, and cartilage breakdown appear in an x-ray of the joint. According to recent statistics, osteoarthritis affects 20 million adults in the U.S. alone.[1]

While osteoarthritis is often given as a diagnosis for pain, evidence supports that it is the result of another painful problem, rather than being the primary cause. As discussed in Chapter 3, osteoarthritis can develop due to instability of a joint that has resulted from trauma or overstretching (relaxation) of a ligament or tendon. In fact, this stretching and injury to the ligament is believed by some medical researchers to be the most important factor in the later development of osteoarthritis.[2] Instability results in a change in the joint's biomechanics, which then creates a change in the wear pattern on the joint, compensation by structures surrounding the weakened joint, and increased stress on the joint. This is especially true for weight-bearing joints such as the knees, hips, or spine.

Remember Wolff's Law, which states: **"Bone responds to stress by making more bone."** Even a slightly unstable joint has more physical stress because now the bones are moving more than they normally would. It doesn't take much extra movement in a joint to create stress. Think of it like the "butterfly effect," where even a slight degree of change can set about a chain of events that alters body mechanics, compensation, and fosters the development of osteoarthritis, pain, and disability.

Medical research on the causes of osteoarthritis has been ongoing for many years. A study done in the Netherlands investigated the correlation between initial ligament damage and the development of subsequent osteoarthritis. This study concluded that a strong relationship exists between the severity of the initial ligament damage and the severity of the osteoarthritis seen later.[3] Another study reviewed the records of individuals who had suffered ligament injury to their knees to see if 12 years later they had developed osteoarthritis. The results of the study were that 63 percent of those people did develop osteoarthritis.[4] A similar study of female soccer players showed a high prevalence of osteoarthritis and x-ray changes in the women who had earlier ligament injury.[5] Animal research has also shown the direct relationship between persistent instability of a joint and later development of osteoarthritis.[6]

Surgery can also cause osteoarthritis later in the joint that had the surgery. The conclusion of one large Swedish study was that patients who underwent meniscetomy (removal of the meniscus in the knee) had a 10- to 18-fold increased likelihood of developing osteoarthritis in the operated knee.[7] This is logical because removing the meniscus makes less room in the joint, while the length of the ligament holding the joint is the same, creating a less stable joint. Remember the body responds to this by building more bone!

If the osteoarthritis gets severe enough it can be a problem in and of itself, especially if it starts affecting joint structure. This is especially true with hips, where, if the degeneration has gone on too long, the hip may need replacement. However, unless the person has a badly degenerated or destroyed joint, Prolotherapy may help—as long as the person is generally healthy. This is because Prolotherapy treats the cause of the problem—ligament and tendon relaxation—by stimulating tissue repair and strengthening. Prolotherapy can help rebuild injured and arthritic joints even years after the initial trauma, by stimulating the production of growth factors.[8] The bony spurs and calcium deposits won't go away, but the amazing thing is that, after Prolotherapy, the pain often improves.[9]

Because joint instability from ligamentous injury is believed to be an important factor in the development of arthritis, wouldn't it be better to prevent arthritis by making sure the joint was completely stable and healed after an injury? If, however, the injury occurred years ago and you are now faced with the diagnosis of "arthritis," Prolotherapy may still be able to help.[10,11]

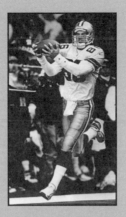

A Professional Football Player

Iplayed quarterback/receiver at University of Washington from 1990 to 1994, tight end for the Dallas Cowboys from 1995 to 1999 and the New England Patriots in 2000. I had a chronic case of turf toe for about six years. It is a really painful injury, and it contributed to pain in my back, knees, and hips due to compensation. I could only wear certain shoes, and it bothered me to walk and while I slept. I had tried all the traditional treatments, including ice, stim, ultrasound, chiropractic, acupuncture, acupressure, orthotics, cortisone shots, and a variety of supplements, with little or no success. I constantly had to use anti-inflammatory medication to play because the pain affected my performance.

My chiropractor suggested I try Prolotherapy. I went through six treatments and have noticed a significant improvement in my condition. It is by far the best my toe has felt in years, and I only wish I had known about Prolotherapy while I was still playing football.

Eric Bjornson
Former Tight End, Dallas Cowboys

CHAPTER 14

Prolotherapy for Sports Injuries

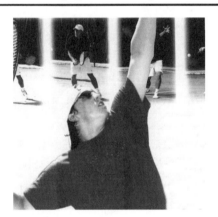

**Gregg Hill, international tennis player,
credits Prolotherapy for saving his career**

Prolotherapy has hit the sports world. It shows up in news reports from time to time in reference to sports injuries and professional athletes. You may also hear it referred to as "injection therapy" or "regenerative injection treatment." Because of the growing demand for Prolotherapy in the sports world, *Prolo Your Sports Injuries Away!* (available from **www.BeulahLandPress.com**) was published in 2001. This excellent resource explains the "hows" and "whys" of Prolotherapy for sports injuries.

Gregg Hill, previously ranked among the top tennis players in the world, has stated that if not for Prolotherapy he wouldn't be playing tennis today.[1] Other sports figures associated in the media and publications with the treatment include Johnnie Morton, former wide receiver for the San Francisco 49ers, Kansas City Chiefs, and Detroit Lions, who credits Prolotherapy for his first pain-free football season in years;[2] Eric Bjornson, former tight end for the Dallas Cowboys and the New England Patriots;[3] David Sloan, former tight end for the New Orleans Saints;[4] and former Mr. Universe Joe DeAngelis.[5]

Also claiming success with Prolotherapy are Stan Mikita, National Hockey League Hall of Famer; Kendall Gill, former NBA Guard for the New Jersey Nets; Lance Dreher, former Mr. Universe; and Ed Fiori, a four-time PGA Tour winner.[6] Recently, Michael Pittman, running back for the Tampa Bay Buccaneers, received Prolotherapy treatment for a severe ankle injury and was able to return to the game much sooner than anticipated.[7]

In the academic world, double-blind studies with professional athletes and Prolotherapy have emerged. A 2005 study looks at Prolotherapy use in elite rugby/soccer players. Out of 24 athletes who chronically could not play at a high level and who failed conservative treatment for groin pain, 20 were pain free and 22 were playing their full sport unrestricted after an average of 2.8 Prolotherapy treatments.[8]

It's no wonder athletes are turning to Prolotherapy—it is a natural treatment that stimulates healing, improves strength, and restores tissue, not to mention its potential to prevent the later development of osteoarthritis. Compare this to cortisone or anti-inflammatory drugs, which cover up the symptoms and weaken tissue.

Regarding Prolotherapy received for his very painful turf toe, recently retired Dallas Cowboy Eric Bjornson writes: "It is by far the best my toe has felt in years, and I only wish I had known about Prolotherapy while I was still playing football" (*Patient Story: A Professional Football Player*, pg. 115). More and more athletes are discovering Prolotherapy before the end of their career, greatly enhancing their professional lives.

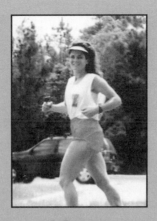

A Runner

Iam an active runner and have been for years. Unfortunately, I had an incredibly unstable ankle that had been sprained over and over again for years, then broke and also dislocated several times while running. I saw an orthopedic surgeon who told me that only surgery could help this condition, but even that wasn't a sure thing. I then heard about Prolotherapy and began to get treatments. Now, after a few months of Prolotherapy treatment, my ankle is incredibly stable and feels stronger than my "good" ankle. I'm running regularly and with no pain or feeling of instability. I'm really, really happy with my result.

Sally Zehnal
Runner

CHAPTER 15

Frequently Asked Questions about Prolotherapy

Does the treatment hurt and is sedation required?

In most cases, no sedation or pain medication is needed. Don't get me wrong, there is some discomfort. A shot is a shot, after all. However, the procedure is well tolerated by most people, as the needles used are thin and the procedure is relatively rapid. I have had some people sing or chat with me during a procedure, while others just grit their teeth. If too uncomfortable, medications can be given such as using a topical anesthetic or a mild pain medication, however 95 percent of the time this is not necessary.

What substances are injected?

Different formulas are used in Prolotherapy, the choice depending upon the doctor's training, the condition being treated, possible patient allergies, and the patient's response to treatment. I primarily use the Hemwall-Hackett-Hauser formula, which is dextrose (a corn extract), Sarapin (a pitcher plant extract), and lidocaine or procaine (numbing agents). Sometimes other ingredients such as zinc, manganese, or morruate (a fish oil extract) are added. Also, a solution called "P2G," which is a combination of dextrose, phenol, and glycerin, may be used. Formulas based on saline and calcium also exist. A starting formula is used and then adjusted, depending on the patient's response to treatment.

How will I feel immediately afterward?

In the first hour or so after a treatment, the pain you came in for may feel like it has decreased. This is because there is a small amount of numbing medication, usually lidocaine, in the formula. If the correct pain triggers are injected with the proliferant solution, those pain triggers are also numbed a little, resulting in some instant pain relief. This does not always happen, however. After the anesthetic wears off, the treated area will generally feel stiff and sore.

How much pain will I be in the next day?

The amount of after-treatment pain varies among patients—a fact I cannot stress enough. All individuals respond to treatment differently, so there is no way to predict exactly what your experience will be. Usually, patients are sore for a day or two and some individuals are very sore. After the initial inflammation and as the body heals, the pain from the treatment improves. I have also seen delayed reactions, where a person feels no pain initially after the treatment and then a few days to a week later experiences a lot of inflammation. I have also seen people experience a lot of pain for about a week or more after treatment, although this is rare. Some people expect a lot of inflammation after treatment and are disappointed if this does not occur. However, there is no need for disappointment. Whether there is a lot of pain after treatment, or none at all, people generally do well. The important thing to remember is to be consistent in your treatments and let your doctor know how you are doing.

What are the reasons for immediate pain relief after a treatment?

Sometimes right after a treatment, the pain goes away completely for a week to several weeks. There are a few possible reasons for this. One is that the injected solution itself along with the initial fluid and inflammation that are induced provide stability to the joint. Another reason is that a "trigger point" may have been released by the injections. Trigger points are painfully tight areas in a muscle where a spasm is occurring. While Prolotherapy injections are not directed to trigger points, inevitably some of them do get injected during the course of treatment, which can be a pleasant side benefit.

Trigger points develop in a muscle after it has been working for a while to hold in a weak joint. The muscle gets "smart" and makes a trigger point so that it can stay tight without as much work. Injecting and releasing trigger points can bring relief in the short term. In fact, trigger point injection therapy is sometimes done alone as a pain treatment and was the basis of the research by Dr. Janet Travel, JFK's personal physician, in the 1950s. But, in general, unless the underlying ligament or tendon is healed, the pain will return with time because the trigger point is usually not the true cause of the problem. Ligament and tendon weakness is! When the ligaments and tendons strengthen and the joint heals, trigger points have a tendency to go away on their own; therefore, they are not usually addressed directly during a Prolotherapy treatment. In some cases, though, trigger points persist after Prolotherapy treatments. I believe this occurs because the body is so used to having these "knots" that it doesn't easily let go of them. If trigger points continue after the joint is repaired, the doctor can then inject them directly.

When will I start noticing improvement?

This, too, varies. I have seen immediate results in some, and in others not until several treatments. On average, I expect some positive changes after the second or third treatment. The reason dramatic improvement does not usually happen on the first treatment is that building new tissue takes time. Just as making a baby takes nine months, healing requires time. No matter how much you want that baby in a week, it's just not going to happen (at least not with our current technology!). So, we wait for the body to make the baby. Similarly, with collagen growth the body needs time to build and repair. If you have been taking pain medication or anti-inflammatory drugs and then stop them to get Prolotherapy treatment, or if you have hypermobile joints, it may take longer for you to notice improvement.

Can Prolotherapy stimulate cartilage repair?

This is a good question. The answer is "maybe"; however, there have not been adequate studies to prove this in the same way that studies have been done regarding ligaments and tendons. Clinically, doctors may see evidence of cartilage regeneration with Prolotherapy, and it is logical to assume Prolotherapy can do this.[1] However, it is important to understand that cartilage has no blood supply whatsoever and thus intrinsically is very difficult tissue to regenerate.[2] Lab research has shown that irritation and mechanical injury to cartilage are necessary to stimulate new cartilage proliferation,[3] so it is logical that if anything could stimulate cartilage to repair, it would be Prolotherapy. Remember, though, that if there is no cartilage left, either because of wear and tear or surgical removal, there is no "seed" to regenerate. However, even if cartilage does not regenerate, improving the strength and stability of surrounding ligaments and tendons has been seen to improve joint stability—reducing or eliminating pain.

How many injections are there in a Prolotherapy treatment?

Prolotherapy treatments involve multiple injections; exactly how many depends on the area(s) being treated. The injections are made at the fibro-osseous junction (*fibro* for "fiber," *osseous* for "bone"). This is the place where ligaments and tendons attach to the bone and growth can be stimulated. To get the best result, the area is peppered with injections. It is difficult to say exactly how many injections a particular person may get during a treatment, but it is more than one injection, and can go up to 50 or more, depending on the areas being treated.

What are the procedure's risks?

While any treatment involving injections has some risk, Prolotherapy is considered low risk. However, the risks that do exist should be thoroughly discussed with your doctor prior to being treated. The most common hazard is bruising. Though bruising can be unsightly and make the area a little more sore, it does not interfere with treatment results. Other risks, though very rare, include infection, allergic reaction, nerve irritation, and puncturing an organ (for example, puncturing the lungs if doing rib injections). There is the risk of being very sore the next day, and feeling worse temporarily. The average length of soreness is a day or two, but could last longer in some cases. Specific risks vary depending on areas being treated and, as in any medical procedure there are unforeseen risks. These risks should all be discussed with your doctor prior to treatment.

On the other hand, there is also the risk—as with any medical procedure—that the treatment won't work. Results can never be guaranteed. Prolotherapy has a strong track record with a high success rate; however, some people simply don't respond to it. (I'd estimate that of the individuals who are appropriate candidates for Prolotherapy treatment, there is a 90 percent success rate with 10 percent not responding.)

What are the reasons Prolotherapy wouldn't work?

Non-responsiveness to treatment has to do with several factors. First is a person's ability to heal. Some people have trouble healing or making new, strong collagen. Other factors that interfere with healing may include medications the person is taking, over-activity resulting in re-injury or re-aggravation of the treatment area, poor nutrition, smoking (which interferes with collagen repair), or severe sleep disturbances. Secondly, Prolotherapy might not work because there was too much damage, such as in the case of a severely degenerated joint, completely ruptured tendon, or bone degeneration, causing the pain. Finally, Prolotherapy might not work if there is something else causing the pain (i.e., it's not really a musculoskeletal problem; for instance, as with an underlying disease process).

What if I am taking anti-inflammatory medication when I begin treatment?

Because Prolotherapy is intended to cause inflammation, you should not be taking anti-inflammatory medication while getting treatment. If you have been taking these types of drugs and wish to begin Prolotherapy, you will be advised to stop the medication prior to treatment. Keep in mind, however, that stopping an anti-inflammatory at the same time as beginning Prolotherapy can be a "double-whammy." The anti-inflammatory medication has been covering up pain in many areas of the body, not just the area being treated. Suddenly off the drug, you may start to feel aches and pains in spots you've never felt before. On top of that, the spot being treated may seem to respond slowly. In this case, it will be more difficult to determine progress in the early stages of treatment.

I recall one particular patient who had been taking 2400 mg of ibuprofen a day—a huge amount. She went "cold turkey" off the medication just before beginning Prolotherapy. After a few treatments, she told me, "Well, I don't notice any difference. I'm in the same amount of pain." So I asked her, "How many ibuprofens are you taking now?" She replied, "None." I said, "Well, there's the difference! You have the same level of pain but without the medication. That is improvement!" She then realized how much better she had become—how much stronger she felt and how much more she was able to do. She continued to do well, requiring only a few more than average total number of treatments. So remember this if you have been taking anti-inflammatories or any other pain medication—and be patient!

What if I am taking a baby aspirin for my heart, or need to take an anti-inflammatory for some other reason?

One baby aspirin a day is too low a dosage to interfere with Prolotherapy. Patients who are taking a higher dose of aspirin or other anti-inflammatory for any reason must be evaluated on an individual basis. In some cases they can undergo Prolotherapy treatment in spite of being on these medications, in other cases not. However, if they do get treatment, it may take longer to see results.

How will I notice improvement?

Improvement shows in different ways. There are objective measurements, such as orthopedic testing done in the doctor's office, which test range of motion and strength and can be rechecked to assess progress. Another important measure of progress, however, is subjective improvement—in other words, how you feel you are doing, how much pain you have been experiencing, and how active you have become. As a person undergoes treatment, he or she will begin to have less pain and to increase activity. Comments I've frequently heard during treatment that indicate subjective improvement are: "I feel stronger," "I have less overall pain," "the joint feels more stable," "I'm able to sit longer," and "I need less pain medication." Sometimes, after initial improvement, some of the original pain feels as though it is coming back, though to a lesser degree. Therefore, the Prolotherapy process can feel like four steps forward, two steps back until the person has completed treatment and is stable.

How many treatments are needed and how often?

While on some occasions I have seen just one or two treatments do the job, this is not the norm. Most often, a person needs between four and six sessions to heal completely. In some cases, more than six may be needed.

Treatments are spaced out according to the doctor's recommendations for the specific problem. Usually treatment is scheduled every four weeks, as this timing works with the body's natural healing cycle. However, the schedule can vary from every six weeks to a more aggressive timeframe of every one, two, or three weeks. The frequency of treatments depends on how well the person heals, as well as his or her normal healing cycle, health status, type of injury, and expected activity level. For professional athletes, for example, the treatment is usually more aggressive because athletes are actively using the body part, are typically very healthy, and tend to have a faster healing cycle. Thus, a 20-year-old athlete could likely be treated much more aggressively than could an 80-year-old great-grandmother.

Why do most people need more than one treatment?

Prolotherapy works by using the body's "stimulus-response" mechanism to heal. The stimulus is the injections; the response, hopefully, is the healing.

I love the way Dr. Ross Hauser describes the reason for multiple treatments: "Doing Prolotherapy is like getting a child to clean his or her room. You may be lucky and it may happen on the first request, but usually it's more like this: First time: 'Clean your room.' Oh, not done … 'Clean your room!' … some work done …'**Clean your room!!!!!**' Most work done…'**CLEAN YOUR ROOM!!**' then the room is finally clean."

So, the idea in Prolotherapy is to get the body to heal by stimulating the areas in need, gentle coaxing, and repetition. While it is rare that a person's pain will resolve in one treatment, it has happened, and did happen to my mother. (See *My Mother's Story*, pg. 141)

Like the turtle and the hare, slow-and-steady progress is the expectation. Of course, while I advise my patients on the usual course, I am happy when they make a faster recovery.

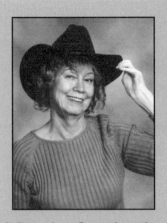

A Dancing Grandmother

I've always been a very active person. I love dancing and used to go dancing five nights per week. I would go square dancing, ballroom dancing, country line dancing, and did jumping jacks every night. I was quite flexible because of being double-jointed, but never had any injuries before. I also raised four children and have several grandchildren. Then, a couple of years ago, I fell and injured my back. I suddenly had to stop all my activity because of the terrible pain in my back and down my leg. I lost a lot of muscle in my legs, couldn't walk, bend, sit, or even lay down without pain. I was told I had a pinched nerve. I wasn't able to dance as I used to and, in fact, had trouble playing with my grandchildren. I saw all kinds of doctors and was told there was nothing that could be done—except perhaps surgery, which I did not want. Then I found out about Prolotherapy. I have had several treatments now, and I'm able to do jumping jacks, dance, and exercise again. The pain is gone!

Jeanne Rosas
Grandmother

CHAPTER 16

Joint Pain: The Diet Connection— Food for Thought

**Let food be thy medicine,
and let thy medicine be food.**

*~ Hippocrates, Father of Medicine
(460–377 BC)*

Food is the one thing we put into our bodies every day, and so it is clearly something that can have an effect on us. In the medical literature, connections have been made between diet and joint pain. The exactness of this connection is not clear. Evidence has shown that certain foods can affect joint pain in some people and that certain supplements may improve or prevent arthritic conditions. However, genetic variations between individuals influence their response to nutritional treatment approaches, and there is controversy around this issue. Yet, because of the magnitude of the problem—70 million American adults are afflicted with some form of joint pain or arthritis[1]—nutrition is a factor that should not be overlooked.

Doctors now think osteoarthritis may begin silently in one's younger years—30s or even 20s—but not show up until much later. Food allergies may be one culprit, as they have been implicated in joint pain.[2,3] A person can be allergic to the foods he or she eats on a regular basis, without showing any obvious symptoms. However, the body can build up antibodies against those foods, which can then form complexes with the foods it sees as "foreign." These complexes can store in the joints, causing pain, sometimes days after eating the offending foods. For that reason, when joint pain persists, testing for food allergies is a good idea.

A particular family of foods known as the "nightshades" (also called the "deadly nightshades") has been recognized for many years to cause debilitating arthritis in animals.[4,5] This family of foods includes tomatoes, potatoes, eggplant, peppers (all kinds except black), and spices such as cayenne, chili, ground red pepper, curry, and paprika. While people are not animals, similar phenomena have been observed in some individuals sensitive to these foods. The nightshade family has been implicated in muscle spasm as well as in joint pain and stiffness.[6] In patient studies, avoiding these foods has resulted in positive to marked improvement in joint pain and arthritis symptoms.[7] While these foods are integrated into much of the American lifestyle and are difficult to avoid, you may want to consider eliminating them from your diet, especially if you are having persistent joint or muscle pain.

What are natural remedies for joint pain? Certainly glucosamine sulfate deserves mention. *The Lancet*, a well-respected medical journal, published a long-term study looking at the effect of glucosamine sulfate to slow the progression of osteoarthritis and in rebuilding bone and cartilage surfaces. The study, done over three years, demonstrated significant improvement in the group taking the supplement at a dose of 1500 mg per day.[8]

In 1962, arthritis research done at the National Institutes of Health brought about the accidental discovery of another effective supplement, a fatty acid named cetyl myrisoleate (CM). A certain type of mouse was found to be resistant to developing arthritis. Further investigation revealed this mouse had something the other lab animals did not—CM.[9] CM was then extracted for use in humans, studied, found to be safe and to offer significant benefit for some, but not all, people with arthritis.[10]

Another arthritis remedy was uncovered when it was noted that coastal-dwelling natives in New Zealand have an extremely low incidence of arthritis as compared to those further inland.[11] The difference between the two was the heavy consumption of the green-lipped mussel by the coastal group. Multiple studies have shown this food to be safe with no real side effects and to decrease pain when compared to placebo,[12] but again may not work for all people.

Still another promising supplement is SAM-e (short for *S-adenosylmethionine*), which comes from the breakdown of the essential amino acid methionine, a protein naturally occurring in foods. Used since the mid-1970s for arthritis, SAM-e also has a positive effect on mood. A 1987 double-blind study of 734 patients including 582 with osteoarthritis of the hip or knee compared using SAM-e to naproxen (an anti-inflammatory medication) and showed that SAM-e was as effective as the anti-inflammatory with fewer side effects.[13] Another double-blind study of patients with osteoarthritis showed SAM-e as effective as ibuprofen (another anti-inflammatory) for reducing pain and increasing mobility.[14]

Finally, Omega-3 Essential Fatty Acids (EFAs), such as salmon oil, have received a lot of positive attention. A recent study compared arthritis patients using Omega-3 EFAs versus those using ibuprofen and demonstrated equivalent effect in reducing arthritic pain.[15] Not only are Omega-3 EFAs a safer alternative to anti-inflammatories, they have been associated with other health benefits such as lower cholesterol[16] and blood pressure,[17] and, most recently, improved cognitive function.[18] Keep in mind, it is important to make sure that if you take this fish oil supplement you get a high-quality brand that is mercury free.

The body uses nutrition to rebuild tissues. Therefore, when getting Prolotherapy, it is important that the right amino acids and collagen-forming nutrients are available in the body. For that reason, I recommend that all my patients take "Prolo Max" by Ortho Molecular, or a similar supplement, while undergoing Prolotherapy. Knox gelatin is also helpful for ensuring the body has enough protein. Similarly, I always encourage my vegetarian patients to take supplemental protein.

As Hippocrates appropriately advised, "Let food be thy medicine." While not the complete answer, nutrition plays a crucial role in healing and should not be overlooked.

MY MOTHER'S STORY

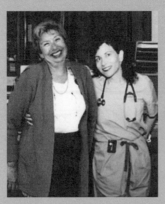

Dr. Alderman with her mother, one happy customer, after Prolotherapy cured her knee pain

I come from a conservative family. My mother, who is an R.N., was extremely skeptical of a non-traditional approach to medicine. In fact, she used to call me the "voodoo doctor." So, when she hurt her knee and became unable to exercise or take her daily walk, I wasn't the first person she called. She consulted an orthopedist, an internist, and a neurologist. She even consulted my brother, who is a kidney doctor. They all told her there was nothing that could be done and that she would just have to live with the pain and stop any aggressive walking or exercising. With a trip to Europe coming up that would involve a lot of walking, my mother became desperate and asked me to "do my voodoo."

I gave her one Prolotherapy treatment on her very painful knee. Two weeks later she called, delighted, and told me, "It's a miracle—the pain is gone!" She went to Europe, had a great time, and was able to walk and enjoy herself without problem. When she got back, she had one more treatment. This was several years ago, and that knee problem did not return. Now she calls me first for her musculoskeletal pain. We recently fixed her plantar fasciitis and she no longer calls me "Doctor Voodoo"!

CHAPTER 17

The Road You Walk

Life is full of choices. Granted, you may not have chosen to be in a motor vehicle accident that left you with years of neck and back pain, or to twist an ankle while playing basketball that never quite healed. But even if you didn't choose your situation, you do have a choice about what to do now. After all, it is *your* body. Far too often we let the medical community tell us what to do, tell us what is best for us. Maybe the advice we get is good, but maybe it isn't. Medical treatment must make sense to you—because you are the one taking the risks. While you cannot always predict the outcome, you can do enough research to make an intelligent decision that seems right for you. Ultimately, what medical treatment you receive is your choice and you will experience the consequences of that choice. Let me tell you about Mike.

Mike walked into my office using a cane, bent over like a thin twig that had been hit hard in a torrid snowstorm. A mere 40 years old, he was ragged and worn from pain and moved like he was 80. He had trouble getting up from a chair, walking for very long, and sitting. Mike told me he had been this way for several months. He experienced terrible low back pain on his left side, which shot down the back of his leg and into his foot. Because of the pain, he often was unable to sleep.

Mike had been to another clinic, where he was prescribed narcotic painkillers just to function. He had started physical therapy, been scheduled for an MRI, and told that he would probably need surgery. Mike worked as a college professor at a local university but, incapable of standing for very long, he had not been able to teach. But what bothered Mike the most was his inability to lift or play with his 6-month-old daughter, Jessica.

After examining Mike and determining that he was a candidate for Prolotherapy, I told him that it was his choice which direction to go. I could see the road he was walking down—one sure to be filled with stronger and stronger painkilling narcotics that would not only lower his immune system, but reduce his mental capacity and clarity as well. And since painkillers do nothing to cure pain—they only temporarily cover it up—these drugs would not heal him. Because depression often accompanies pain and a diminished way of life, Mike would probably be prescribed anti-depressants at some point as well. But the anti-depressants wouldn't solve the problem either. Mike was walking down a road filled with these mind-weakening drugs, more pain, and then likely a surgery that he might not need but would be desperate enough to undergo.

Don't get me wrong—sometimes people do need surgery. Far too often, however, the surgeon relies on the MRI for his diagnosis, and, as you know by now, MRIs are not acceptable evidence that surgery is needed. As you will recall from Chapter 8, abnormal findings on MRIs in people with low back pain might be coincidental and not the actual cause of their pain.[1] Time and time again in my practice, I have found this to be true.

An MRI needs to be correlated to the individual. To simply look at the MRI and say, "This disc is herniated, so it must be the problem. Let's cut it out," will not resolve the problem if the problem is not the disc. And because I have seen patients who have undergone multiple surgeries for back pain that did not resolve the pain, I consider surgery a last resort unless it is truly indicated.

Mike was a conservative guy, brought up to respect authority, and wanted to follow his other doctor's advice for the time being. He said he would think about his options and would come back if he wanted to try Prolotherapy. I did not see Mike again for several months, until one day he showed up for an appointment. I was shocked to see how much worse he had become. He had almost doubled his intake of painkillers and reported that, in spite of everything, he was still in constant pain and unable to work. He had been told he needed surgery, but had been putting it off. He asked for my help, and we started Prolotherapy treatments that day. Three months later he was walking without a cane, and six months later he was playing and lifting

Jessica, now a toddler. Mike had gone back to work and was able to stop taking painkillers. The day I "graduated" him from treatment he practically danced out of the office, happy and smiling. And he never did have that surgery.

This story may not be yours, for truly every experience is different. However, the bottom line is that each of us has a choice of which road to walk, and when to walk it. I hope this book has been useful to you in your journey. Well wishes to you, on whatever road you choose!

Appendix
Prolotherapy Studies, Research Articles, and Books

- Ahn, K.H., H.S. Kim, et al. "The Effect of Prolotherapy on the Injured Achilles Tendon in a Rat Model." *J. Korean Acad. Rehabil. Med.* (June 2002) 26, no. 3: 332–6. Korean.

- Alderman, D. "Prolotherapy for Musculoskeletal Pain." *Practical Pain Management* (Jan/Feb 2007): 10–15.

- Alderman, D. "Prolotherapy for Low Back Pain." *Practical Pain Management* (May 2007): 58–63.

- Alderman, D. "Prolotherapy for Knee Pain." *Practical Pain Management* (July/August 2007): 70–79.

- Banks, A.R. "A Rationale for Prolotherapy." *Journal of Orthopaedic Medicine* 13, no. 3 (1991).

- Blaschke, J.A. "Conservative Management of Intervertebral Disk Injuries." *Journal of the Oklahoma State Medical Association* 54, no. 9 (1961).

- Blumenthal, L.S. "Injury to the Cervical Spine as a Cause of Headache." *Postgraduate Medicine* 56, no. 3 (1974).

- Borenstein, D.G., S.W. Wiesel, and S.D. Boden, editors. *Low Back Pain: Medical Diagnosis and Comprehensive Management.* 2nd ed. Philadelphia, PA: W.B. Saunders Co., 1995.

- Brody, J. "Injections to Kickstart Tissue-Repair." *The New York Times.* Health Section (August 7, 2007): D8.

- Bronston, G.J. "Injection Therapy for Ligamentous Strain." *Journal of the National Association of Chiropodists* 47, no. 12 (1957).

- Bronston, G.J. "The Strengthening of Chronically Strained Ankle Ligaments with Injections of Sodium Psylliate." *Journal of the American Podiatry Association* 48, no. 11 (1959).

- Chase, R.H. "Basic Sclerotherapy." *Osteopathic Annals* 6, no. 12 (1978): 16–20.

- Clayton, M.I., and G.J. Weir. "Experimental Investigations of Ligamentous Healing." *American Journal of Surgery* 98 (1959): 373–8.

- Conti, G.V. "The Unstable Low Back: Causes and Treatment." *Osteopathic Annals* 6, no. 12 (1978): 36–41.

- Cyriax, J., and G. Russell. *Textbook of Orthopaedic Medicine: Vol. 2. Treatment by Manipulation, Massage and Injection.* 9th ed. Baltimore, MD: Williams & Wilkins.

- Cyriax, J. *Textbook of Orthopaedic Medicine: Vol. 1. Diagnosis of Soft Tissue Lesions.* 8th ed. London, UK: Bailliere Tindall.

- Darrow, M. *The Collagen Revolution: Living Pain Free.* Los Angeles, CA: Protex Press, 2002.

- Darrow, M. *Prolotherapy: The Hollywood Pain Solution.* Los Angeles, CA: Protex Press, 2003.

- Daum, W.J. "The Sacroiliac Joint: An Underappreciated Pain Generator." *The American Journal of Orthopedics* (June 1995).

- Dechow, E., R.K. Davie, et al. "A Randomized, Double-Blind, Placebo-Controlled Trial of Sclerosing Injections in Patients with Chronic Low Back Pain." *Rheumatology* 38, no. 12 (1999): 1255–9.

- Dorman, T.A., editor. *Spine: Prolotherapy in the Lumbar Spine and Pelvis.* Philadelphia, PA: Hanley & Belfus, Inc., 1995.

- Dorman, T.A., and T.H. Ravin. *Diagnosis and Injection Techniques in Orthopedic Medicine.* Baltimore, MD: Williams & Wilkins, 1991.

- Dorman, T.A. "Back Pain, a Misunderstood, Often Misdiagnosed 20th Century Scourge." *Fact, Fiction & Fraud in Modern Medicine* 1, no. 4 (1996).

- Dorman, T.A. "Introducing Prolotherapy and Orthopedic Medicine." *Fact, Fiction & Fraud in Modern Medicine* 1, no. 5 (1996).

- Dorman, T.A. "Prolotherapy: A Survey." *The Journal of Orthopaedic Medicine* 15, no. 2 (1993): 49–50.

- Dussault, R.G., and P.A. Kaplan. "Facet Joint Injection: Diagnosis and Therapy." *Applied Radiology* (June 1994).

- Faber, W.J. "Biological Reconstruction—Alternative to Hip Prosthesis." *Health Freedom News* (June 1990).

- Faber, W.J. "Biological Reconstruction: Solution for Refractory Head and Neck Pain." *The Journal of Neurological & Orthopaedic Medicine & Surgery* 12 (1991): 6–11.

- Faber, W.J. "Non-Surgical Tendon, Ligament and Joint Reconstruction." *Townsend Letter for Doctors* (May 1993).

- Faber, W.J., and M. Walker. *Pain, Pain Go Away.* ISHI Press International, 1990.

- Frost, Jr., W.W. "Case Study: Sacro-iliac Problems and the Benefit of Prolotherapy Over Time." *The Journal of Orthopaedic Medicine* 16, no. 3 (1994).

- Green, S. "The Study of Ligamentous Tissue Is Regarded as Key to Sclerotherapy." *The Osteopathic Profession* (January 1958).

- Greenman, P.E. *Principles of Manual Medicine*. 2nd ed. Baltimore, MD: Williams & Wilkins, 1996.

- Gross, L. "An Innovative Solution for Aching Joints?" *Muscle and Fitness* (January 2002): 92–8.

- Hackett, G.S., G.A. Hemwall, and G.A. Montgomery. *Ligament and Tendon Relaxation Treated by Prolotherapy*. 5th ed. Oak Brook, IL: Institute in Basic Life Principles, 1991.

- Hackett, G.S., and D.G. Henderson. "Joint Stabilization." *American Journal of Surgery* 89 (1955): 968–73.

- Hackett, G.S., T.C. Huang, and A. Raftery. "Prolotherapy for Headache, Pain in the Head and Neck and Neuritis." *Headache* (April 1962).

- Hackett, G.S. *Ligament and Tendon Relaxation Treated by Prolotherapy*. 3rd ed. Springfield, IL: Charles C. Thomas, 1958.

- Hackett, G.S. "Low Back Pain." *The British Journal of Physical Medicine* 19, no. 2 (1956): 25–35.

- Hackett, G.S. "Prolotherapy of Sciatica from Weak Pelvic Ligaments and Bone Dystrophy." *Clinical Medicine* 8, no. 12 (1961).

- Hackett, G.S. "Shearing Injury to the Sacroiliac Joint." *The Journal of the International College of Surgeons* 22, no. 6 (1954).

- Harris, F.I., A.S. White, and G.R. Bisking. "Observations on Solutions Used for Injection Treatment of Hernia." *American Journal of Surgery* 39 (1938): 112–9.

- Hauser, R., and M. Hauser. *Prolo Your Pain Away!* Oak Park, IL: Beulah Land Press, 1998.

- Hauser, R., and M. Hauser, et al. *Prolo Your Sports Injuries Away!* Oak Park, IL: Beulah Land Press, 2001.

- Hauser, R., and M. Hauser. *Prolotherapy: An Alternative to Knee Surgery.* Oak Park, IL: Beulah Land Press, 2004.

- Hauser, R., and M. Hauser. "Dextrose Prolotherapy for Unresolved Neck Pain." *Practical Pain Management* (October 2007).

- Hauser, R., and M. Hauser, and K. Blakemore. "Dextrose Prolotherapy for Tempomandibular Joint Dysfunction." *Practical Pain Management* (December 2007).

- Helfet, A.J., D.M. Gruebel Lee, et al. *Disorders of the Lumbar Spine.* Philadelphia, PA: J.B. Lippincott Co.

- Hirschberg, G.G., L. Froetscher, and F. Naeim. "Iliolumbar Syndrome as a Common Cause of Low Back Pain: Diagnosis and Prognosis." *Archives of Physical Medicine and Rehabilitation* 60 (1979).

- Howes, R.G., and I.C. Isdale. "The Loose Back: An Unrecognized Syndrome." *Rheumatology and Physical Medicine* 11, no. 2 (1971).

- Jo, D., and M. Kim. "Effects of Prolotherapy on Knee Joint Pain Due to Ligament Laxity." *Korean J. Pain* (June 2004) 17, no. 1: 47–50. Korean.

- Jo, D., K. Ryu, et al. "The Effects of Prolotherapy on Shoulder Pain." *Korean J. Anesthesiology* (May 2004) 46, no. 5: 589–92. Korean.

- Jo, D.H., S.J. Yang, et al. "The Effects of Prolotherapy on the Lumbar Herniated Nucleus Pulposus." *Korean J. Pain* (June 2003) 16, no. 1: 68–72. Korean.

- Kang, S.H., K.M Seo, et al. "Ultrasonographic Findings of Chronic Lateral Epicondylititis with Partial Tear Before and After Prolotherapy." *J. Korean Acad. Rehabil. Med.* (February 2004) 28, no. 1: 88–93. Korean.

- Kayfetz, D.O., L.S. Blumenthal, et al. "Whiplash Injury and Other Ligamentous Headache—Its Management with Prolotherapy." *Headache* 3, no. 1 (1963).

- Kayfetz, D.O. "Occipito-cervical (Whiplash) Injuries Treated by Prolotherapy." *Medical Trial Technique Quarterly* (June 1963).

- Kim, B.K., J.Y. Shin, et al. "The Effect of Prolotherapy for the Chronic Pain of Musculoskeletal System." *J. Korean Acad. Rehabil. Med.* (February 2001) 25, no. 1: 128–33. Korean.

- Kim, H.J., S.H. Kim, et al. "The Effects of Anti-inflammatory Drugs on Histologic Findings of the Experimental Prolotherapy Model." *J. Korean Acad. Rehabil. Med.* (August 2006) 30, no. 4: 378–84. Korean.

- Kim, H.J., T.S. Jeong, et al. "Comparison of Histological Changes in Accordance with the Level of Dextrose-Concentration in Experimental Prolotherapy Model." *J. Korean Acad. Rehabil. Med.* (December 2003) 27, no. 6: 935–40. Korean.

- Kim, H.S., K.H. Ahn, et al. "Comparison Between the Effect of Local Steroid Injection and Prolotherapy on Iliac Crest Pain Syndrome." *J. Korean Acad. Rehabil. Med.* (February 2007) 31, no. 1: 20–4. Korean.

- Kim, J.M. "The Effect of Prolotherapy for Osteoarthritis of the Knee." *J. Korean Acad. Rehabil. Med.* (August 2002) 26, no. 4: 445–8. Korean.

- Kim, S.A., E.H. Kim, et al. "The Effects of Hyperosmolar Dextrose and Autologous Serum Injection in the Experimental Articular Defect of Rabbit." *J. Korean Acad. Rehabil. Med.* (April 2006) 30, no. 2: 173–8. Korean.

- Kim, S.H., Y.H. Jeon, et al. "Effects of Prolotherapy on Chronic Musculoskeletal Disease." *Korean J. Pain* (December 2002) 15, no. 2: 121–5. Korean.

- Klein, R.G., T.A. Dorman, and C.E. Johnson. "Proliferant Injections for Low Back Pain, Histologic Changes of Injected Ligaments and Objective Measurements of Lumbar Spine Mobility Before and After Treatment." *The Journal of Neurological & Orthopaedic Medicine & Surgery* 10, no. 2 (1989).

- Klein, R.G., B.C. Eek, et al. "A Randomized Double-Blind Trial of Dextrose-Glycerinephenol Injections for Chronic, Low Back Pain." *Journal of Spinal Disorders* 6, no. 1 (1993): 23–33.

- Koudele, C.J. "Treatment of Joint Pain." *Osteopathic Annals* 6, no. 12 (1978).

- Lee, C.W., Y.S. Kim, et al. "Clinical Experience of Prolotherapy for Chronic Musculoskeletal Disease: A Report of 5 Cases." *Korean J. Pain* (June 2001) 14, no. 1: 114–7. Korean.

- Leedy, R.F. "Applications of Sclerotherapy to Specific Problems." *Osteopathic Medicine* (September 1977): 79–81, 85–95.

- Leedy, R.F. "Basic Techniques of Sclerotherapy." *Osteopathic Medicine* (August 1977): 17–22, 189–44.

- Liu, Y.K., C.M. Tipton, et al. "An In-situ Study of the Influence of a Sclerosing Solution in Rabbit Medial Collateral Ligaments and Its Junction Strength." *Connective Tissue Research* 11, no. 23 (1983); 95–102.

- Manoil, L. "Histologic Effects of Various Sclerosing Solutions." *Archives of Surgery* 36, no. 2 (1938): 171–89.

- Maynard, J.A., V.A. Pedrini, et al. "Morphological and Biochemical Effects of Sodium Morrhuate on Tendons." *Journal of Orthopaedic Research* 3 (1985): 236–48.

- Merriman, J.R. "Prolotherapy Versus Operative Fusion in the Treatment of Joint Instability of the Spine and Pelvis." *Journal of the International College of Surgeons* 42, no. 2 (1964): 150–9.

- Mooney, V. "Prolotherapy at the Fringe of Medical Care, or Is It the Frontier?" *Spine* 3, no. 4 (July/August 2003): 253.

- Myers, A. "Prolotherapy Treatment of Low Back Pain and Sciatica." *Bulletin of the Hospital for Joint Diseases* 11, no. 1 (1961).

- Naeim, F., L. Froetscher, and G.G. Hirschberg. "Treatment of the Chronic Iliolumbar Syndrome by Infiltration of the Iliolumbar Ligament." *The Western Journal of Medicine* 136, no. 4 (1982).

- Ombregt, L., P. Bisschop, et al, eds. *A System of Orthopaedic Medicine.* London, UK: W.B. Saunders Co. Ltd., 1995.

- Ongley, M.J., T.A. Dorman, et al. "Ligament Instability of Knees: A New Approach to Treatment." *Manual Medicine* 3 (1988): 152–4.

- Ongley, M.J., R.G. Klein, et al. "A New Approach to the Treatment of Chronic Low Back Pain." *The Lancet* (July 1987): 143–6.

- Park, J.H., I.S. Song, et al. "Ultrasonographic Findings of Healing of Torn Tendon in the Patients with Lateral Epicondylitis After Prolotherapy." *J. Korean Soc. Med. Ultrasound* (September 2003) 22, no. 3: 177–83. Korean.

- Park, J.Y. "Nonsurgical Management of Chronic Low Back Pain." *J. Korean Med. Assoc.* (June 2007) 50, no. 6: 507–22. Korean.

- Reeves, K.D., and K.M. Hassanein. "Long-term Effects of Dextrose Prolotherapy for Anterior Cruciate Ligament Laxity: A Prospective and Consecutive Patient Study." *Alternative Therapies in Health and Medicine* 9, no. 3 (2003): 58–62.

- Reeves, K.D., and K.M. Hassanein. "Randomized Prospective Double-blind Placebo-controlled Study of Dextrose Prolotherapy for Knee Osteoarthritis with or without ACL Laxity." *Alternative Therapie in Health and Medicines* 6, no. 2 (2000): 68–79.

- Reeves, K.D., and K.M. Hassanein. "Randomized, Prospective, Double-blind Placebo-controlled Study of Dextrose Prolotherapy for Osteoarthritic Thumb and Finger (DIP, PIP and Trapeziometacarpal) Joints: Evidence of Clinical Efficacy." *Journal of Alternative and Complementary Medicine* 6, no. 4 (2000): 311–20.

- Reeves, K.D. "Prolotherapy: Basic Science, Clinical Studies, and Technique. In *Pain Procedures in Clinical Practice.* 2nd ed. Lennard, T.A. (editor). Philadelphia, PA: Hanley and Belfus, 2000.

- Reeves, K.D. "Prolotherapy, Present and Future Applications in Soft-tissue Pain and Disability. Injection Techniques: Principles and Practice." *Physical Medicine and Rehabilitation* 6, no. 4 (1995): 917–26.

- Reeves, K.D. "Sweet Relief." *Biomechanics* (September 2004): 25–35.

- Reeves, K.D. "Technique of Prolotherapy." In *Physiatric Procedures.* Lennard, T.A. (editor). Philadelphia, PA: Hanley & Belfus, Inc., 1995.

- Reeves, K.D. "Treatment of Consecutive Severe Fibromyalgia Patients with Prolotherapy." *Journal of Orthopaedic Medicine* 16, no. 3 (1994).

- Rice, C.O., and H. Mattson. "Histologic Changes in the Tissues of Man and Animals Following the Injection of Irritating Solutions Intended for the Cure of Hernia." *Illinois Medical Journal* (September 1936): 271–8.

- Schultz, L.W. "Treatment for Subluxation of the Temporomandibular Joint." *Journal of the American Medical Association* (September 1937).

- Schultz, L.W. "Twenty Years: Experience in Treating Hypermobility of the Temporomandibular Joints." *American Journal of Surgery* 92 (1956).

- Schwartz, R.G., and N. Sagedy. "Prolotherapy: A Literature Review and Retrospective Study." *The Journal of Neurological and Orthopedic Medicine and Surgery* 12, no. 3 (1991): 220–3.

- Shin, J.Y., K.M. Seo, et al. "The Effect of Prolotherapy on Lateral Epicondylitis of Elbow." *J. Korean Acad. Rehabil. Med.* (December 2002) 26, no. 6: 764–8. Korean.

- Shuman, D., guest editor. "Sclerotherapy." *Osteopathic Annals* 1978; 6(12): 10–4.

- Shuman, D. "Ambulation, Osteopathic Manipulative Therapy and Joint Sclerotherapy in the Management of Common Low-Back Disorders." *Journal of the American Osteopathic Association* 67 (1967).

- Topol, G.A., K.H. Reeves, and K. Hassanein. "Efficacy of Dextrose Prolotherapy in Elite Male Kicking-Sport Athletes with Chronic Groin Pain." *Archives of Physical Medicine and Rehabilitation* 86 (2005): 697–702.

- Vanderschot, L. "The American Version of Acupuncture: Prolotherapy: Coming to an Understanding." *American Journal of Acupuncture* 4, no. 4 (1976).

- Vleeming, A., V. Mooney, et al, eds. *Movement, Stability and Low Back Pain: The Essential Role of the Pelvis.* New York, NY: Churchill Livingstone, 1997.

- Walmer, H.C. "A Comprehensive, Nonsurgical Approach to the Low-Back Problem." *Osteopathic Annals* 6, no. 12 (1978): 29–34.

- Willman, W.S. "Solutions Employed in Sclerotherapy." *Osteopathic Annals* 6, no. 2 (1978): 519–21.

- Yelland, M.J., P.P. Glaszious, et al. "Prolotherapy Injections, Saline Injections, and Exercises for Chronic Low-Back Pain: A Randomized Trial." *Spine* 29, no. 1 (2004): 9–16.

- Zimmerman, J. "Sacro-iliac Joint Dysfunction." *Physical Therapy Forum* (October 1991).

Notes

Chapter 1

[1] Blue Shield of California, *Evidence of Coverage and Health Service Agreement*, February 2005, Part I: DEFINITIONS, 7.

[2] State of California, *Business and Professions Code*, Section 2453(a), Article 21, 2003.

[3] College of Osteopathic Medicine of the Pacific. "Osteopathic Medical History and Philosophy." http://www.westernu.edu/comp/omm_history.xml.

Chapter 2

[1] Andriacchi, T., P. Sabiston, K. DeHaven, et al. "Ligament: Injury and Repair." *Acta Rheum Scand.* 1956; 2:109-116.

[2] Reeves, K.D. "Prolotherapy: Basic science, clinical studies and technique." In Lennard, T.A. (editor). *Pain Procedures in Clinical Practice.* 2nd ed. Philadelphia, PA: Hanley and Belfus, 2000; 172-190.

[3] Reeves, K.D. "Prolotherapy: Basic Science, clinical studies and technique." In *Pain Procedures in Clinical Practice.* 2nd ed. Philadelphia, PA: Hanley and Belfus, 2000.

[4] Liu, Y. "An in-situ study of the influence of a sclerosing solution in rabbit medial collateral ligaments and its junction strength." *Connective Tissue Research.* 1983; 2:95-102.

[5] Maynard, J. "Morphological and biomechanical effects of sodium Morrhuate on tendons." *Journal of Orthopaedic Research.* 1985; 3:236-248.

[6] Klein, R. "Proliferant injections for low back pain: Histologic changes of injected ligaments and objective measures of lumbar spine mobility before and after treatment." *Journal of Neurology, Orthopedic Medicine and Surgery.* 1989; 10:141-144.

[7] Reeves, K.D., and K. Hassanein. "Randomized prospective double-blind placebo-controlled study of dextrose Prolotherapy for knee osteoarthritis with or without ACL laxity." *Alternative Therapies*. March 2000; 6(2):68-80.

[8] Otsuka Y., H. Mizuta, K. Takagi, et al. "Requirement of fibroblast growth factor signaling for regeneration of epiphyseal morphology in rabbit full-thickness defects of articular cartilage." *Dev Growth Differ*. 1997; 39:143-156.

[9] Van Beuningen, H., H. Glansbeek, P. van der Kraan, et al. "Differential effects of local application of BMP-2 or TGF-beta 1 on both articular cartilage composition and osteophyte formation." *Osteoarthritis Cartilage*. 1998; 6:306-317.

[10] C. Everett Koop. Preface in Hauser, *Prolo Your Pain Away!* Oak Park, IL: Beulah Land Press, 1998, 15-17.

Chapter 3

[1] Hauser, R., and M. Hauser. *Prolo Your Pain Away!* Oak Park, IL: Beulah Land Press, 1999.

[2] Hackett, G.S., G.A. Hemwall, and G.A. Montgomery. *Ligament and Tendon Relaxation Treated by Prolotherapy*. 5th ed. Oak Brook, IL: Institute in Basic Life Principles, 1991.

[3] Alpers, B.J. "The problem of sciatica." *Medical Clinics of North America*. 1953; 37:503.

[4] Hackett, G.S., G.A. Hemwall, and G.A. Montgomery. *Ligament and Tendon Relaxation Treated by Prolotherapy*. 5th ed. Oak Brook, IL: Institute in Basic Life Principles, 1991.

[5] Hackett, G.S., and D.G. Henderson. "Joint stabilization: an experimental, histologic study with comments on the clinical application in ligament proliferation." *American Journal of Surgery*. 1955; 80:968-973.

[6] Alpers, B.J. "The problem of sciatica." *Medical Clinics of North America.* 1953; 37:503.

[7] Hackett, G.S., G.A. Hemwall, and G.A. Montgomery. *Ligament and Tendon Relaxation Treated by Prolotherapy.* 5th ed. Commenting on work of P.H. Newman. Oak Brook, IL: Institute in Basic Life Principles, 1991, 9.

[8] Morehead, K., and K. Sack. "Osteoarthritis: What therapies for this disease of many causes?" *Postgraduate Medicine.* November 2003:12-17.

[9] Lohmander, L.S., A. Ostenberg, M. Englund, and H. Roos. "High prevalence of knee osteoarthritis, pain and functional limitations in female soccer players twelve years after anterior cruciate ligament injury." *Arthritis & Rheumatism.* October 2004; 50(10):3142-3152.

[10] Panush, R. "Recreational activities and degenerative joint disease." *Sports Medicine.* January 1994; 17:1-5.

[11] Farrow, C.S., and C.D. Newton. "Ligamentous Injury (Sprain)." In *Textbook of Small Animal Orthopaedics.* Ithaca, NY: International Veterinary Information Service, 1985.

[12] Morehead, K., and K. Sack. "Osteoarthritis: What therapies for this disease of many causes?" *Postgraduate Medicine.* November 2003:12-17.

[13] Cervoni, T.D., et al. "Recognizing upper-extremity stress lesions." *The Physician and Sportsmedicine.* August 1997; 25:8.

[14] Linetsky, F.S., K. Botwin, L. Gorfine, et al. Position Paper: "Regenerative injection therapy (RIT) effectiveness and appropriate usage." The Florida Academy of Pain Medicine, May 24, 2001. http://www.aaomed.org/library/documents/RIT_Position_Paper_052301.pdf

[15] Reeves, K.D., and K. Hassanein. "Randomized prospective doubleblind placebo-controlled study of dextrose prolotherapy for knee osteoarthritis with or without ACL laxity." *Alternative Therapies.* March 2000; 6(2):68-79.

[16] Reeves, K.D., and K. Hassanein. "Randomized prospective placebo controlled double blind study of dextrose prolotherapy for osteoarthritic thumbs and finger (DIP, PIP and Trapeziometacarpal) joints: Evidence of clinical efficacy." *Journal of Alternative and Complementary Medicine.* 2000; 6(4):311-320.

[17] *Taber's Cyclopedic Medical Dictionary.* 18th ed. s.v. "collagen." F.A. Davis Company, 1997, 411.

[18] Banks, A.R. "A Rationale for Prolotherapy." *Journal of Orthopaedic Medicine.* 1991; 13(3).

[19] Stovitz, S.D., and R.J. Johnson. "NSAIDs and musculoskeletal treatment: what is the clinical evidence?" *The Physician and Sportsmedicine.* 2003; 31:1.

[20] Reeves, K.D. "Prolotherapy: Basic Science, Clinical Studies, and Technique." In Lennard, T.A. (editor). *Pain Procedures in Clinical Practice.* 2nd ed. Philadelphia, PA: Hanley and Belfus, 2000, 172-190.

[21] Reeves, K.D., and K. Hassanein. "Randomized prospective double-blind placebo-controlled study of dextrose Prolotherapy for knee osteoarthritis with or without ACL Laxity." *Alternative Therapies.* 2000; 6:68-80.

[22] Dagenais, S., S. Haldeman, and J.R. Wooley. "Intraligamentous injection of sclerosing solutions (prolotherapy) for spinal pain: a critical review of the literature." *The Spine Journal.* 2005; 5:310-328.

[23] Reeves, K.D. "Prolotherapy: Basic Science, Clinical Studies, and Technique." In Lennard, T.A. (editor). *Pain Procedures in Clinical Practice.* 2nd ed. Philadelphia, PA: Hanley and Belfus, 2000, 172-190.

[24] Reeves K.D. "Prolotherapy: Present and Future Applications in Soft-Tissue Pain and Disability. Injection Techniques: Principles and Practice." *Physical Medicine and Rehabilitation Clinics of North America.* November 1995; 6(4):917-923.

Chapter 4

[1] "Alternative treatments: Dealing with chronic pain." *Mayo Clinic Health Letter.* April 2005; 23(4).

[2] Hauser, R., and M. Hauser, et al. *Prolo Your Sports Injuries Away!* Oak Park, IL: Beulah Land Press, 2001, xi.

[3] Hauser, R., and M. Hauser, et al. *Prolo Your Sports Injuries Away!* Oak Park, IL: Beulah Land Press, 2001.

[4] Schnirring, L. "News Brief: Are your patients asking about Prolotherapy?" *The Physician and Sportsmedicine.* 28(8):15-17.

[5] Reeves, K.D., and K. Hassanein. "Randomized prospective double-blind placebo-controlled study of dextrose Prolotherapy for knee osteoarthritis with or without ACL laxity." *Alternative Therapies.* March 2000; 6(2):68-80.

[6] Liu, Y.K., C.M. Tipton, R.D. Matthes, et al. "An in situ study of the influence of a sclerosing solution in rabbit medial collateral ligaments and its junction strength." *Connective Tissue Research.* 1983; 11:95-102.

[7] Maynard, J.A., et al. "Morphological and biochemical effects of sodium morrhuate on tendons." *Journal of Orthopaedic Research.* 1985; 3:236-248.

[8] Reeves, K.D. "Randomized, prospective, placebo-controlled double-blind study of dextrose Prolotherapy for osteoarthritic thumb and finger (DIP, PIP, and trapeziometacarpal) joints: Evidence of clinical efficacy." *The Journal of Alternative and Complementary Medicine.* November 2000; 6(4):311-320.

[9] Reeves, K.D. "Treatment of consecutive severe fibromyalgia patients with Prolotherapy." *The Journal of Orthopaedic Medicine*. 1994; 16(3):84-89.

[10] Liu, Y.K., C.M. Tipton, R.D. Matthes, et al. "An in situ study of the influence of a sclerosing solution in rabbit medial collateral ligaments and its junction strength." *Connective Tissue Research*. 1983; 2:95-102.

[11] Liu, Y.K., C.M. Tipton, R.D. Matthes, et al. "An in situ study of the influence of a sclerosing solution in rabbit medial collateral ligaments and its junction strength." *Connective Tissue Research*. 1983; 2:95-102.

[12] Maynard, J.A., et al. "Morphological and biochemical effects of sodium morrhuate on tendons." *Journal of Orthopaedic Research*. 1985; 3:326-248.

[13] Klein, Dorman, and Johnson. "Proliferant injections for low back pain: Histologic changes of injected ligaments & objective measurements of lumbar spine mobility before and after treatment." *The Journal of Neurological & Orthopaedic Medicine & Surgery*. 1989; 10:141-144.

[14] The Florida Academy of Pain Medicine. "Position paper on regenerative injection therapy: Effectiveness and appropriate usage." May 24, 2001. In *The Pain Clinic Magazine*. June 2002; 4(3):38-45. Also on http://www.aaomed.org/library/documents/RIT_Position_Paper_052301.pdf.

[15] Klein, R.G., J. Patterson, B. Eek, and D. Zeiger. "Prolotherapy for the Treatment of Back Pain." *American Association of Orthopedic Medicine Position Statement*. http://www.aaomed.org/library/documents/Prolo_position_back_pain.pdf.

[16] Hooper, R.A., and M. Ding. "Retrospective case series on patients with chronic spinal pain treated with dextrose Prolotherapy." *Journal of Alternative and Complementary Medicine*. August 2004; 10(4):670-674.

[17] Hackett, G. "Joint stabilization: An experimental, histologic study with comments on the clinical application in ligament proliferation." *American Journal of Surgery*. May 1955; 89:968-973. Quoted in Hauser, R., et al, *Prolo Your Sports Injuries Away!* Oak Park, IL: Beulah Land Press, 2001, 30.

[18] Hauser, R. "The research of Gustav A. Hemwall." Prolotherapy Chicagoland Chronic Pain and Sports Specialists. http://www. prolonews.com/ how_safe_is_prolotherapy.htm.

Chapter 5

[1] Reeves, K.D. "Prolotherapy: Basic Science, Clinical Studies, and Technique." In Lennard, T.A. (editor). *Pain Procedures in Clinical Practice*. 2nd ed. Philadelphia, PA: Hanley and Belfus, 2000, 166.

Chapter 6

[1] Faber, W.J., and M. Walker. *Pain, Pain Go Away*. Ishi Press International, 1990.

[2] Saberski, L. *Preface* in *Prolo Your Sports Injuries Away!* Oak Park, IL: Beulah Land Press, 2001.

[3] Brody, J. "Injections to Kick Start Tissue Repair." *NY Times* Personal Health Section, August 7, 2007, D8.

Chapter 7

[1] Hackett, G.S., G.A. Hemwall, and G.A. Montgomery. *Ligament and Tendon Relaxation Treated by Prolotherapy*. 5th ed. Oak Brook, IL: Institute in Basic Life Principles, 1991, xxv.

Chapter 8

[1] Ombregt, Bisschop, and ter Veer. *A System of Orthopaedic Medicine*. 2nd ed. Churchill Livingstone, 2003, 59.

[2] MacRae, D.L. "Asymptomatic intervertebral disc protrusion." *Acta Radiologica*. 1956; 46-49.

[3] Hitselberger, W.E., and R.M. Whitten. "Abnormal myelograms in asymptomatic patients." *Journal of Neurosurgery*. 1968; 28:204.

[4] Wiesel, S.W., et al. "A study of computer-assisted tomography: 1. The incidence of positive CAT scans in an asymptomatic group of patients." *Spine.* 1984; 9:549-551.

[5] Powell, M.C., et al. "Prevalence of lumbar disc degeneration observed by magnetic resonance in symptomless woman." *Lancet.* 1986; 13:1366-1367.

[6] Boden, S.D., et al. "Abnormal magnetic resonance scans of the lumbar spine in asymptomatic subjects." *Journal of Bone and Joint Surgery.* 1990; 72A:503-408.

[7] Kaplan, P.A. "MR imaging of the normal shoulder: Variants and pitfalls." *Radiology.* 1992; 184:519-524.

[8] Deyo, R. "Magnetic resonance imaging of the lumbar spine— terrific test or tar baby?" *New England Journal of Medicine.* 1994; 331:115-116.

[9] Matsumoto, M., et al. "MRI of the cervical intervertebral discs in asymptomatic subjects." *Journal of Bone and Joint Surgery* (Br). 1998; 80(1):19-24.

[10] Humphreys, S.C., et al. "Reliability of magnetic resonance imaging in predicting disc material posterior to the posterior longitudinal ligament in the cervical spine, a prospective study." *Spine.* 1998; 23(22):2468-2471.

[11] Kaiser, J.A., and B.A. Holland. "Imaging of the cervical spine." *Spine.* 1998; 23(24):2701-2712.

[12] Jerosch, J., W.H. Castro, and J. Assheuer. "Age related magnetic resonance imaging morphology of the menisci in asymptomatic individuals." *Archives of Orthopedic Trauma Surgery.* 1996; 115(3-4);199-202.

[13] LaPrade, R.F., et al. "The prevalence of abnormal magnetic resonance imaging findings in asymptomatic knees. With correlation of magnetic resonance imaging to arthroscopic findings in symptomatic knees." *American Journal of Sports Medicine.* 1994; 22(6):739-745.

[14] Stanitski, C.L. "Correlation of arthroscopic and clinical examinations with magnetic resonance imaging findings of injured knees in children and adolescents." *American Journal of Sports Medicine.* 1998; 26:2-6.

[15] Chandnani, V., et al. "MR findings in asymptomatic shoulders: A blind analysis using symptomatic shoulders as controls." *Clinical Imaging.* 1992; 16:25-30.

[16] Sher, J.S., et al. "Abnormal findings on magnetic resonance images of asymptomatic shoulders." *Journal of Bone and Joint Surgery.* 1995; 75A:10-15.

[17] Miniaci, A., et al. "Magnetic resonance imaging evaluation of the rotator cuff tendons in the asymptomatic shoulder." *American Journal of Sports Medicine.* 1995; 23:142-145.

[18] Thompson, W.O., et al. "A biomechanical analysis of rotator cuff deficiency in a cadaveric model." *American Journal of Sports Medicine.* 1996; 24(3):286-292.

[19] Miniaci, A., et al., "Magnetic imaging of the shoulder in asymptomatic professional baseball pitchers." *American Journal of Sports Medicine.* 2002; 20:66-73.

[20] Connor, P.M., et al. "Magnetic resonance imaging of the asymptomatic shoulder of overhead athletes: A 5-Year Follow-up Study." *American Journal of Sports Medicine.* 2003; 31:724-727.

[21] Ibid.

[22] Moseley, J. Bruce, et al. "A controlled trial of arthroscopic surgery for osteoarthritis of the knee for osteoarthritis of the knee." *The New England Journal of Medicine.* July 11, 2002; 347(2):81-88.

[23] Borenstein, D.G. "Etiology of low back pain." *Family Practice Recertification.* 1999; 2(7), (Suppl.): 3-7.

Chapter 9

[1] Loh, Roy S. "Effects of opioids on the immune system." *Neurochem Res.* November 1996; 21(11):1375-1386.

[2] Stovitz, S.D., and R.J. Johnson. "NSAIDs and musculoskeletal treatment. What is the clinical evidence?" *The Physician and Sportsmedicine.* January 2003; (31)1.

[3] Juni, P., et al. "Risk of cardiovascular events and Rofecoxib [Vioox]: cumulative meta-analysis." *The Lancet.* December 2004; 364(9450): 2021-2029.

[4] Welters, I. "Opioids and immunosuppression. Clinical relevance?" *Anaesthesist.* May 2003; 52(5):442-452.

[5] Loh, R.S. "Effects of opioids on the immune system." *Neurochem Res.* November 1996; 21(11):1375-1386.

[6] Sacerdote, P., et al. "The effects of tramadol and morphine on immune responses and pain after surgery in cancer patients." *Anesth Analg.* June 2000; 90(6):1411-1414.

[7] Zhang, N., et al. "Ca+2- independent protein kinase C's mediate heterologous desensitization of leukocyte chemokine receptors by opioid receptors." *Journal of Biological Chemistry.* April 11, 2003; 278(15):12729-12736.

[8] Scopsi, L., et al. "Immunoreactive opioid peptides in human breast cancer." *American Journal of Pathology.* 1989; 134(2):473-479.

[9] Simon, R.H., and T.E. Arbo. "Morphine increases metastatic tumor growth." *Brain Research Bulletin.* 1986; 16(3):363-367.

[10] Ishikawa, M., et al. "Enhancement of tumor growth by morphine and its possible mechanism in mice." *Biol Pharm Bull.* 1993; 16(3):762-766.

[11] Bryan, H., et al. "Immunosuppressive effects of chronic morphine treatment in mice." *Life Science.* 1987; 41(14):1731-1738.

[12] Stovitz, S.D., and R.J. Johnson. "NSAIDs and musculoskeletal treatment. What is the clinical evidence?" *The Physician and Sportsmedicine.* January 2003; 31(1).

[13] Golden, B.D., and S.D. Abramson. "Selective cyclooxygenase-2 inhibitors." *Rheumatology Clinics of North America.* 1999; 25(2):359-278.

[14] Segev, G., and R. Katz. "Selective COX-2 inhibitors and risk of cardiovascular events." *Hospital Physician.* February 2004; 39-46.

[15] Elder, C.L., L.E. Dahners, and P.S. Weinhold. "A cyclooxygenase-2 inhibitor impairs ligament healing in the rat." *The American Journal of Sports Medicine.* 2001; 29(6):801-805.

[16] Stovitz, S.D., and R.J. Johnson. "NSAIDs and musculoskeletal treatment. What is the clinical evidence?" *The Physician and Sportsmedicine.* January 2003; 31:1.

[17] Ibid.

[18] Orchard, J., and T. Best. "The management of muscle strain injuries: An early return versus the risk of recurrence." *Clinical Journal of Sports Medicine.* 2002; 12(1):3-5.

[19] Almekinders, L.C., and J.A. Gilbert. "Healing of experimental muscle strains and the effects of nonsteroidal anti-inflammatory medication." *American Journal of Sports Medicine.* 1986; 14:303-308.

[20] Misra, D., et al. "Anti-inflammatory medication after muscle injury." *Journal of Bone and Joint Surgery.* 1995; 77:1510-1519.

[21] Obremsky, W., et al. "Biomechanical and histologic assessment of a controlled muscle strain injury treated with piroxicam." *American Journal of Sports Medicine.* 1994; 22:558-561.

[22] Stovitz, S.D., and R.J. Johnson. "NSAIDs and musculoskeletal treatment. What is the clinical evidence?" *The Physician and Sportsmedicine.* January 2003; 31(1).

[23] Ibid.

[24] Almekinders, L.C. "Anti-inflammatory treatment of muscular injuries in sports." *Sports Medicine.* 1993; 15:139-145.

[25] Slatyer, M.A., M.J. Hensley, and R. Lopert. "A randomized controlled trial of Piroxicam in the management of acute ankle sprain in Australian Regular Army recruits: The Kapooka Ankle Sprain Study." *American Journal of Sports Medicine.* 1997; 25(4):544-553.

[26] Elder, C., et al. "A Cox-2 inhibitor impairs ligament healing in the rat." 47th Annual Meeting, Orthopaedic Research Society, February 25-28, 2001, San Francisco, California, and *The American Journal of Sports Medicine.* 2001; 29(6):801-805.

[27] Stanley, K.L., and J.E. Weaver. "Pharmacologic management of pain and inflammation in athletes." *Clinics in Sports Medicine.* 1998; 17(2):374-392.

[28] Almekinders, L.C. "Anti-inflammatory treatment of muscular injuries in sports: An update of recent studies." *Sports Medicine.* 1999; 28(6):383-388.

[29] Glassman, D.S., et al. "The effect of postoperative nonsteroidal anti-inflammatory drug administration on spinal fusion." *Spine.* 1998; 23(7):834-838.

[30] Giannoudis, P.V., et al. "Nonunion of the femoral diaphysis: The influence of reaming and non-steroidal anti-inflammatory drugs." *Journal of Bone and Joint* (Br). March 2001; 83(2):308.

[31] Simon, A.M., et al. "Cyclo-Oxygenase 2 function is essential for bone fracture healing." *Journal of Bone and Mineral Research.* 2002; 17(6):963.

[32] Einhorn, T.A. "Editorial: Do inhibitors of Cyclooxygenase-2 impair bone healing?" *Journal of Bone and Mineral Research.* 2002; 17(6):977-978.

[33] Khan, K.M., et al. "Overuse tendinosis, not tendonitis. Part 1: A new paradigm for a difficult clinical problem." *The Physician and Sportsmedicine.* 2000; 28(5):38-48.

[34] MacFarlane, L.L., et al. "NSAIDs, antihypertensive agents and loss of blood pressure control." *American Family Physician.* 1995; 51(4):849-856.

[35] Vitting, K.E., et al. "Naproxen and acute renal failure in a runner, letter." *Annals of Internal Medicine.* 1986; 105(1):144.

[36] Walker, R.J., et al. "Indomethacin potentiates exercise-induced reduction in renal hemodynamics in athletes." *Medicine and Science in Sports and Exercise.* 1994; 26(11):1302-1306.

[37] Perneger, T.V., et al. "Risk of kidney failure associated with the use of acetaminophen, aspirin and nonsteroidal anti-inflammatory drugs." *The New England Journal of Medicine.* December 1994; 331(25):1675-1679.

[38] Wolfe, M.M., et al. "Gastrointestional toxicity of nonsteroidal anti-inflammatory drugs." *New England Journal of Medicine.* 1999; 340(24):1888-1899. [Published erratum, *New England Journal of Medicine* 1999; 341(7):548)].

[39] ACR 68th Annual Scientific Meeting regarding the Adenomatous Polyp Prevention on Vioxx (APPROVe) trial, presented October 18, 2004.

[40] Segev, G., and R. Katz. "Selective COX-2 inhibitors and risk of cardiovascular events." *Hospital Physician.* February 2004; 39-46.

[41] Stovitz, S.D., and R.J. Johnson. "NSAIDs and musculoskeletal treatment. What is the clinical evidence?" *The Physician and Sportsmedicine.* January 2003; 31(1).

[42] From "NSAIDs: What you need to know." *Arthritis: Self-Management.* July/August 2004, 26.

Chapter 10

[1] Frymoyer, J.W., and W.L. Cats-Baril. "An overview of the incidences and costs of low back pain." *Orthopedic Clinics of North America.* 1991; 22:263-271.

[2] Valkenburg, H.A., and H.C.N. Haanen. "The epidemiology of low back pain." In: White, A.A., and S.L. Gordon (eds). *Idiopathic Low Back Pain.* St. Louis, MO: Mosby, 1982.

[3] Biering-Sorensen, F. "A prospective study of low back pain in general population. I. Occurrence, recurrence and aetiology." *Scandinavian Journal of Rehabilitation Medicine.* 1983; 15:71.

[4] Frymoyer, J.W., and W.L. Cats-Baril. "An overview of the incidences and costs of low back pain." *Orthopedic Clinics of North America.* 1991; 22:263-271.

[5] Hills, E.C., with J. Michael Wieting, et al., eds. "Mechanical low back pain." November 21, 2004. http://www.emedicine.com/pmr/topic73.htm.

[6] Drezner, J., and S. Herring. "Managing low-back pain." *The Physician and Sportsmedicine.* 2001; 29:8.

[7] Ombregt, Bisschop, and ter Veer. *A System of Orthopaedic Medicine.* 2nd ed. Churchill Livingstone, 2003, 700.

[8] Ibid.

[9] Borenstein, D.G. "Chronic low back pain." *Rheumatological Disease Clinics of North America.* 1996; 22:439-456.

[10] Braddom, R.L. "Perils and pointers in the evaluation and management of back pain." *Seminars in Neurology.* 1998; 18:197-210.

[11] Ombregt, Bisschop, and ter Veer. *A System of Orthopaedic Medicine.* 2nd ed. Churchill Livingstone, 2003, 53.

[12] *Stedman's Concise Medical Dictionary.* 4th ed. s.v. "chronic." U.S. National Center for Health Statistics, Lippincott Williams & Wilkins Publishers, 2001, 185.

[13] Ombregt, Bisschop, and ter Veer. *A System of Orthopaedic Medicine.* 2nd ed. Churchill Livingstone, 2003, 739.

[14] Hills, E.C., with J. Michael Wieting, et al, eds. "Mechanical Low Back Pain," November 21, 2004. http://www.emedicine.com/pmr/topic73.htm.

[15] Ombregt, Bisschop, and ter Veer. *A System of Orthopaedic Medicine.* 2nd ed. Churchill Livingstone, 2003, 775.

[16] Mixter, W.J., and J.S. Barr. "Rupture of the intervertebral disc with involvement of the spinal canal." *New England Journal of Medicine.* 1934; 211:210.

Chapter 11

[1] Hakelius, A. "Prognosis in sciatica: A clinical follow-up of surgical and nonsurgical treatment." *Acta Orthopaedica Scandinavica.* 1970; (Suppl): 129.

[2] Nashold, B.S., and Z. Hrubec. *Lumbar Disc Disease: A Twenty-year Clinical Follow-up Study.* St. Louis, MO: Mosby, 1971.

[3] Alaranta, H. "A prospective study of patients with sciatica." *Spine.* 1990; 15:1345-1349.

[4] Bush, K., et al. "The natural history of sciatica associated with disc pathology." *Spine.* 1992; 17:1205-1222.

[5] Delauche-Cavalier, M.C., et al. "Lumbar disc herniation; computed tomography scan changes after conservative treatment of nerve root compression." *Spine.* 1992; 17:927-933.

[6] Matsubara, Y., et al. "Serial changes on MRI in lumbar disc herniations treated conservatively." *Neuroradiology.* 1995; 37:378-383.

[7] Naylor, A. "Intervertebral disc prolapse and degeneration: The biomechanical and biophysical approach." *Spine.* 1976; 1:108.

[8] Hills, E.C., with J. Michael Wieting, et al, eds. "Mechanical low back pain." November 21, 2004. http://www.emedicine.com/pmr/topic73.htm.

[9] Ombregt, Bisschop, and ter Veer. *A System of Orthopaedic Medicine.* 2nd ed. Churchill Livingstone, 2003, 747, 765.

[10] Nachemson, A. "Advances in low back pain." *Clin. Orthop.* 1985; 200:266.

[11] Paster, R.Z. "Nonpharmacologic management of low back pain." *Family Practice Recertification Management of Chronic Low Back Pain Special Supplement.* June 1999; 21(7):6.9-21.

[12] Alpers, B.J. "The problem of sciatica." *Medical Clinics of North America.* 1953; 37:503.

[13] Ombregt, Bisschop, and ter Veer. *A System of Orthopaedic Medicine.* 2nd ed. Churchill Livingstone, 2003, 729.

[14] Hackett, G.S., G.A. Hemwall, and G.A. Montgomery. *Ligament and Tendon Relaxation Treated by Prolotherapy.* 5th ed. Commenting on work of P.H. Newman. Oak Brook, IL: Institute in Basic Life Principles, 1991, 9.

[15] Acarpglu, E.R., et al. "Degeneration and aging affect the tensile behavior of human lumbar annulus fibrosus." *Spine.* 1995; 20:2690-2701.

[16] Krag, M.H., et al. "Thoracic and lumbar internal disc displacement distribution from in vitro loading of human spinal motion segments: experimental results and theoretical predictions." *Spine.* 1987; 12:1001-1007.

[17] Ombregt, Bisschop, and ter Veer. *A System of Orthopaedic Medicine.* 2nd ed. Churchill Livingstone, 2003, 745.

[18] Buschbacher, R. *Practical Guide to Musculoskeletal Disorders: Diagnosis and Rehabilitation.* 2nd ed. Boston, MA: Butterworth Heinemann, 2002, 100.

[19] Ibid.

[20] Cyriax, J.H. *Illustrated Manual of Orthopaedic Medicine.* 2nd ed. Oxford, England: Butterworth-Heineman, 1998, 199.

[21] Merriman, J. "Prolotherapy versus operative fusion in the treatment of joint instability of the spine and pelvis." *Journal of the International College of Surgeons.* August 1964; 42(2):150-159.

[22] Borenstein, D. "Etiology of low back pain." *Family Practice Recertification Management of Chronic Low Back Pain Special Supplement.* June 1999; 21(7):6.

Chapter 12

[1] Frank, C., et al. "Normal ligament properties and ligament healing." *Clin Orthop.* 1985; 15-25.

[2] Almekinders, L., and J. Temple. "Etiology, diagnosis, and treatment of tendonitis: An analysis of the literature." *Medicine & Science in Sports & Exercise.* August 1998; 30(8):1183-1190.

[3] Khan, K.M., et al. "Editorial: Time to abandon the 'tendonitis' myth." *British Medical Journal.* March 2002; 324:626-627.

[4] Maffulli, N., K.M. Khan, and G. Puddu. "Overuse tendon conditions: Time to change a confusing terminology." *Arthroscopy.* 1998; 14:840-843.

[5] Khan, K.M., et al. "Overuse tendonosis, not tendonitis." *The Physician and Sportsmedicine.* 2000; 28(5).

[6] Khan, K.M., et al. "Histopathology of common overuse tendon conditions: Update and implications for clinical management." *Sports Medicine.* 1999; 27:393-408.

[7] Almekinders, L., and J. Temple. "Etiology, diagnosis, and treatment of tendonitis: An analysis of the literature." *Medicine & Science in Sports & Exercise.* August 1998; 30(8):1183-1190.

[8] Liu, Y. "An in situ study of the influence of a sclerosing solution in rabbit medial collateral ligaments and its junction strength." *Connective Tissue Research.* 1983; 2:95-102.

[9] Maynard, J. "Morphological and biomechanical effects of sodium morruhuate on tendons." *Journal of Orthopaedic Research.* 1985; 3:236-248.

[10] Klein, R. "Proliferant injections for low back pain: Histologic changes of injected ligaments and objective measures of lumbar spine mobility before and after treatment." *Journal of Neurology, Orthopedic Medicine and Surgery.* 1989; 10:141-144.

[11] Reeves, K.D. and K. Hassanein. "Randomized prospective double-blind placebo-controlled study of dextrose Prolotherapy for knee osteoarthritis with or without ACL laxity." *Alternative Therapies.* March 2000; 6(2):68-80.

Chapter 13

[1] National Institutes of Health, National Institute of Arthritis and Musculsokeletal and Skin Diseases, "Arthritis Prevalence Rising as Baby Boomers Grow Older; Osteoarthritis Second Only to Chronic Heart Disease in Worksite Disability" [press release]. May 5, 1998. http://www.niams.nih.gov/ne/press/05_05.htm.

[2] Lowman, E. "Osteoarthritis." *Journal of the American Medical Association.* 1955; 157:487-488.

[3] Van Osch, G.M., et al. "Relation of ligament damage with site specific cartilage loss and osteophyte formation in collagenase induced osteoarthrthritis in mice." *Journal of Rheumatology.* July 1996; 23(7):1227-1232.

[4] Segawa, H., et al. "Long-term results of non-operative treatment of anterior cruciate ligament injury." *The Knee.* March 2001; 8(1):5-11.

[5] Lohmander, L.S., et al. "High prevalence of knee osteoarthritis, pain and functional limitations in female soccer players twelve years after anterior cruciate ligament injury." *Arthritis & Rheumatism.* October 2004; 50(10):3145-3152.

[6] Farrow, C.S., and C.D. Newton. "Ligamentous injury (sprain)." In *Textbook of Small Animal Orthopaedics.* Newton, C.D., and D.M. Nunamaker (eds.). Ithaca, NY: International Veterinary Information Service, 1985.

[7] Brunk, D. "Meniscetomy Associated with Knee Osteoarthritis." *Family Practice News.* February 15, 2006; 50.

[8] Reeves, K.D., and K. Hassanein. "Randomized prospective double-blind placebo-controlled study of dextrose prolotherapy for knee osteoarthritis with or without ACL laxity." *Alternative Therapies.* March 2000; (6)2:68-80.

[9] Reeves, K.D., and K. Hassanein. "Randomized, prospective, placebo-controlled, double-blind study of dextrose prolotherapy for osteoarthritis thumb and finger (DIP, PIP and trapeziometacarpal) joints: Evidence of clinical efficacy." *The Journal of Alternative and Complementary Medicine.* 2000; (6)4:311-320.

[10] Reeves, K.D., and K. Hassanein. "Randomized prospective double-blind placebo-controlled study of dextrose prolotherapy for knee osteoarthritis with or without ACL laxity." *Alternative Therapies.* March 2000; (6)2:68-80.

[11] Reeves, K.D., and K. Hassanein. "Randomized, prospective, placebo-controlled, double-blind study of dextrose prolotherapy for osteoarthritis thumb and finger (DIP, PIP and trapeziometacarpal) joints: Evidence of clinical efficacy." *The Journal of Alternative and Complementary Medicine.* 2000; (6)4:311-320.

Chapter 14

[1] Hauser, R. *Prolotherapy: An Alternative to Knee Surgery.* Oak Park, IL: Beulah Land Press, 2004, vii-ix.

[2] Gross, L. "An innovative solution for aching joints?" *Muscle & Fitness.* January 2002; 92-96.

[3] See his Patient Story on page 115 of this book.

[4] Gross, L. "An innovative solution for aching joints?" *Muscle & Fitness.* January 2002; 92-96.

[5] Goodstein, E. "Breakthrough therapy relieves chronic pain without surgery or drugs." *The National Enquirer.* January 20, 2004; 48.

[6] Hauser, R., et al. *Prolo Your Sports Injuries Away!* Oak Park, IL: Beulah Land Press, 2004.

[7] Holder, S. *The St. Petersburg Times.* November 15, 2007. http://www.bucpower.com/graham1511.html.

[8] Topol, G.A., K.D. Reeves, and K. Hassanein. "Efficacy of dextrose prolotherapy in elite male kicking-sport athletes with chronic groin pain." *Archives Physical Medicine and Rehabilitation.* 2005; 86:697-702.

Chapter 15

[1] Hauser, R., and M. Hauser. *Prolo Your Pain Away!* 2nd ed. Oak Park, IL: Beulah Land Press, 2004, 154.

[2] Newman, A.P. "Articular cartilage repair." *The American Journal of Sports Medicine* 1998; 26:209-324.

[3] Mankin, H.J. "The response of articular cartilage to mechanical injury." *Journal of Bone and Joint Surgery.* 1982; 64(3):460-466.

Chapter 16

[1] Bolen, J., et al. National Center for Chronic Disease Prevention and Health Promotion, CDC. "Prevalence of self-reported arthritis or chronic joint symptoms among adults – United States 2001." *Morbidity and Mortality Weekly Report.* October 25, 2002; 51(42):948-950.

[2] Sampson, H.A. "Food allergy." *Journal of the American Medical Association.* 1997; December 10; 278(22):1888-1894.

[3] Van de Laar, M.A., and J.K. van de Korst. "Food intolerance in rheumatoid arthritis: A double blind controlled trial of the clinical effects of elimination of milk allergens and azo dyes." *Annuals of Rheumatological Diseases*. March 1992.

[4] Lynd, F.T., et al. "The Naalehu disease (in Hawaii)." *American Journal of Veterinary Research*. 1965; 26:1344-1349.

[5] Krook, L., et al. "Cestrum diurnum poisoning in Florida cattle." *Cornell Vet*. 1975; 65(10):557-575.

[6] Childers, N.F., and M.S. Margoles. "An apparent relation of nighshades (solanaceae) to arthritis." *Journal of Neurological and Orthopedic Medical Surgery*. 1993; 12:227-231.

[7] Childres, N.F. *Arthritis-Childer's Diet to Stop It: Nightshades, Aging and Ill Health*. 4th ed. Florida: Horticultural Publications, 1993.

[8] Reginster, J.Y., et al. "Long-term effects of glucosamine sulphate on osteoarthritis progression: A randomized, placebo-controlled clinical trial." *The Lancet*. 2001; 357:251-256.

[9] Diehl, H.W., and E.L. May. "Cetyl myristoleate isolated from Swiss albino mice: an apparent protective agent against adjuvant arthritis in rat." *Journal of Pharmaceutical Science*. 1994; 83:296-299.

[10] Siemandi, H., et al. "Arthritic episodes in patients with various auto-immune diseases characterized by the common terminology 'arthritis' and 'psoriasis': A randomized clinical trial." *Townsend Letter*. Second quarter, 1997.

[11] Whitehouse, M.V., et al. "Anti-inflammatory activity of a lipid fraction (Lyprinol) from the NZ green-lipped mussel." *Inflammopharmacology*. 1997; 5:237-246.

[12] Lau, C.S., et al. "Treatment of knee osteoarthritis with Lyprinol®, lipid extract of the green-lipped mussel—a double-blind placebo-controlled study." *Progress in Nutrition*. 2004.

[13] Caruso, I., and V. Pietrogrande. "Italian double-blind muticenter study comparing S-adenosylmethionine, naproxen and placebo in the treatment of degenerative joint disease." *American Journal of Medicine.* 1987; 83(5A):66-71.

[14] Muller-Fassbender, H. "Double-blind clinical trial of S-adenosylmethionine versus ibuprofen in the treatment of osteoarthritis." *American Journal of Medicine.* 1987; 83(5A):81-83.

[15] Maroon, J., J. Bost, J. Baughman, and M. Wert. Department of Neurosurgery, University of Pittsburgh. "Results of Omega-3 EFA for Spine Pain. Presented at the *American Association Neurological Surgeons Annual Meeting,* New Orleans, April 18, 2005.

[16] Phillipson, F.E., D.W. Rothrock, et al. "Reduction of plasma lipis, lipoproteins, and apoproteins by dietary fish oils in patients with hypertriglyceridemia. *New England Journal of Medicine.* 1985; 312:1210-1216.

[17] Appel., L.J., E.R. Miller, et al. "Does supplementation of diet with 'fish oil' reduce blood pressure? A meta analysis of controlled clinical trials." *Archives of Internal Medicine.* Jan-Feb 1994; 120 (Suppl): 8-10.

[18] Issa, A.M., and W.A. Mojica. "The efficacy of omega-3 fatty acids on cognitive function in aging and dementia: a systematic review." *Dement Geriatr Cogn Disord.* 2006; 21(2):88-96.

Chapter 17

[1] Jensen, M. "Magnetic resonance imaging of the lumbar spine in people without back pain." *New England Journal of Medicine.* 1994; 331:69-73.

Glossary

[1] Day, B., et al. "The vascular and nerve supply of the human meniscus." *Arthroscopy.* 1985; 1(1):58-62.

[2] Hackett, G.S., G.A. Hemwall, G.A. Montgomery. *Ligament and Tendon Relaxation Treated by Prolotherapy*. 5th ed. Oak Brook, IL: Institute in Basic Life Principles, 1991, xix.

[3] *Webster's Third New International Dictionary, Unabridged*. s.v. "prolotherapy." http://unabridged.merriam-webster.com.

[4] Reeves, K.D. "Prolotherapy: Basic science, clinical studies and technique." *Pain Procedures in Clinical Practice*. Hanley & Belfus, Inc., 2000.

[5] Reeves, K.D. "Prolotherapy: Present and Future Applications in Soft Tissue Pain and Disability. Injection Techniques, Principles and Practice." *Physical Medicine and Rehabilitation Clinics of North America*. November 1995; 6(4):917-923.

[6] Ombregt, Bisschop, and ter Veer. *A System of Orthopaedic Medicine*. 2nd ed. Churchill Livingstone, 2003, 59.

Glossary

Cartilage: A firm, dense tissue that provides padding between bones. Cartilage can withstand considerable tension and pressure. However, this tissue has *no* blood or nerve supply of its own and therefore heals poorly.

Cartilage—Articular Cartilage: The type of cartilage that lines the ends of bones in joints is known as "articular cartilage" because it is on the surface of the bones that compose a joint (*articulate* from Latin meaning "to divide").

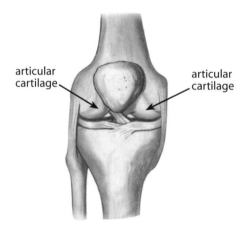

articular cartilage

articular cartilage

Collagen: The most abundant protein in mammals. Collagen is the main component of ligaments, which hold bones together, and also of tendons, which support the joints and provide motion (from Greek *koila*, "glue" and *-gen*, "producing").

Connective Tissue: Tissue that provides support and connection between different parts of the body framework. These tissues include, among other things, ligaments and tendons.

Disc: A flat, round pad of cartilage that sits between two vertebrae in the spine. The disc's purpose is to provide cushioning. The vertebrae-disc units are held together by ligament tissue. The disc has no blood supply of its own and relies on surrounding circulation for any nutrition. Therefore, discs do not regenerate well when injured.

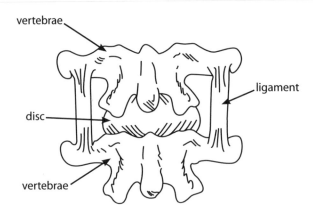

Joint: A joint is where two bones come together to provide motion. Examples include the elbow, shoulder, hip, as well as the individual segments in the neck and back.

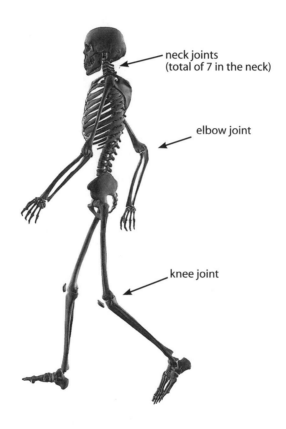

neck joints
(total of 7 in the neck)

elbow joint

knee joint

Ligament: A strong, fibrous material that binds one bone to another in a joint, providing stability to that joint. The tissue is a whitish color, demonstrating poor blood supply.

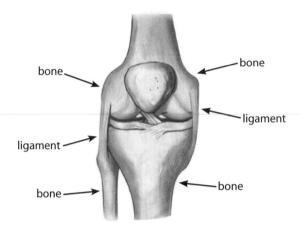

Knee Joint

Ligaments have some flexibility; however, if over-stretched, they may sustain injury, similar to a rope that becomes frayed or torn if pulled too hard.

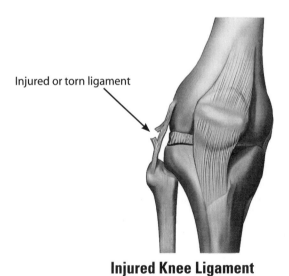

Injured Knee Ligament

Meniscus: A special type of cartilage that sits between the bones of the knee joint, providing cushioning. The meniscus is another tissue with a poor blood supply, receiving only a limited amount to the outer one-third of its structure. Therefore, it does not heal well when injured. There is no blood or nerve supply in the inner two-thirds of the meniscus.[1]

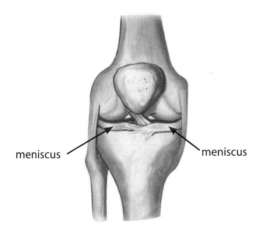

meniscus   meniscus

Prolotherapy: Prolotherapy is a method of injection treatment designed to stimulate healing.[2] It is also known as "proliferant injection therapy," "regenerative injection therapy," and "non-surgical ligament reconstruction." It has been described as "the rehabilitation of an incompetent structure (as a ligament or tendon) by the induced proliferation (growth, repair) of new cells."[3] The word comes from Latin, meaning "to grow progeny, offspring." Prolotherapy has been practiced in the United States since the 1930s.

Sclerotherapy: An older, inaccurate term for Prolotherapy based on the original theory that the treatment worked by producing scar tissue. However, biopsy studies have not demonstrated scar formation with solutions currently in use.[4] Rather, studies have shown new, normal, thicker, and stronger connective tissue after Prolotherapy injections.[5]

Soft Tissue: "Soft tissue" refers to tissue that connects, supports, or surrounds the organs and bones of the body. Soft tissue includes ligaments, tendons, muscle, fat, nerves, and cartilage. Soft tissue injury surrounding a joint causes pain at a moving part of the body. If such injuries do not heal completely, chronic pain can result. According to a well-known orthopedic textbook, soft tissue injuries are thought to be a major cause of human suffering.[6]

Sprain: Overstretching of a ligament that results in injury to a ligament is called a "sprain." The degree of sprain can vary from small micro-tears to complete tears or rupture. An example is a sprained ankle after twisting. This can cause joint laxity (looseness, instability) if the ligament does not heal completely.

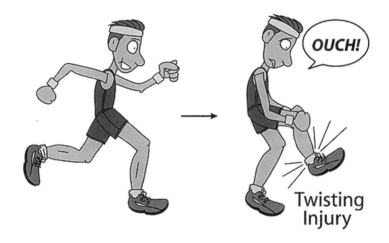

Strain: A "strain" is overstretching of a muscle or tendon. As with sprains, in strains the degree of injury can vary from small micro-tears to rupture. A sprain and strain commonly exist together in the same injury, hence the term *sprain/strain*.

Tendon: The end portion of a muscle that attaches that muscle to a bone, helping provide motion. Tendon tissue is very similar to that of ligaments. Like ligaments, tendons can be overstretched, creating tears and microtears, resulting in pain and weakness.

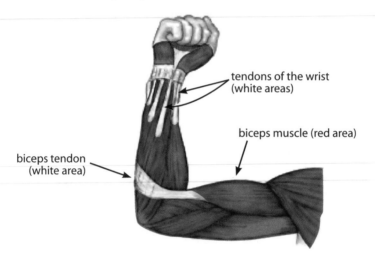

tendons of the wrist (white areas)

biceps muscle (red area)

biceps tendon (white area)

Vertebra (plural is vertebrae): One of the small bones that make up the spine. These bones extend all the way from the top of the neck to the bottom of the tailbone. There is a joint between each set of vertebrae, allowing motion such as bending and turning. Vertebrae are divided into 7 neck vertebrae ("cervical"), 12 mid and upper back vertebrae ("thoracic"), and 5 low back ("lumbar") vertebrae, as well as a tailbone ("sacrum").

Photo/Illustration Credits

Photograph Credits

Photograph on page xiii is courtesy of Ross A. Hauser, M.D.; photographs on page xvii, xix, 60, and 141 are courtesy of the author; photograph on page 1 is courtesy of John Gray, Ph.D.; photograph on page 5 is courtesy of the American Osteopathic Association; photograph on page 9 is courtesy of Jane Edwards; photograph on page 21 is courtesy of Antonia Lattin; photograph on page 35 is courtesy of Joseph Spair; photograph on page 43 is courtesy of Kathy Moore; photograph on page 51 is courtesy of Diana (Shipman) Hamar; photograph on page 57 is courtesy of Jeff Confenti; photograph on page 62 is courtesy of Shawn Ingallina; photograph on page 65 is courtesy of Dawn Derenski; photograph on page 71 is courtesy of Jennifer Freitas; photograph on page 83 is courtesy of Bob Dillon; photograph on page 91 is courtesy of Dann Shubin; photograph on page 103 is courtesy of Brenda Falvi; photograph on page 109 is courtesy of Doug Stokes; photograph on page 115 is courtesy of Eric Bjornson; photograph on page 117 is courtesy of Gregg Hill; photograph on page 121 is courtesy of Sally Zehnal; photograph on page 133 is courtesy of Jeanne Rosas.

Illustration Credits

Illustrations on pages 12, 16, 94, 183, 184, 186 (top), 186 (bottom), 187, and 190 are by Publication Services, Inc.; illustrations on pages 14, 98, and 189 are by Genny

May-Montt; illustrations on pages 18, 30, 47, and 48 are reproduced by permission from Ross A. Hauser and Marion A. Hauser, *Prolo Your Pain Away!* (Oak Park, IL: Beulah Land Press, 2004); illustration on page 100 is courtesy of PPM Communications; illustration on page 135 is by istockphotos.com; illustration on page 185 is by LifeART.

Index

Index

www.prolotherapy.com